DISCUSSIONS OF UNUSUAL TOPICS IN FIBROMYALGIA

Edited by **William S. Wilke**

Discussions of Unusual Topics in Fibromyalgia
http://dx.doi.org/10.5772/66578
Edited by William S. Wilke

Contributors
Emine Eda Kurt, Fatmanur Aybala Koçak, Lucindo José Quintans-Júnior, Renan Guedes Brito, Priscila Laise Santos, Jullyana de Souza Siqueira Quintans, Jackson Roberto Guedes da Silva Almeida, Marlange Almeida Oliveira, Angelo Antoniolli, Gokhan Zengin, Laurent Picot, Licia Pina, Alejandra Guillermina Guillermina Miranda Miranda Díaz, Simón Quetzalcóatl Rodríguez Lata, William S. Wilke

Published by InTech
Janeza Trdine 9, 51000 Rijeka, Croatia

Publishing Process Manager Dajana Pemac
Technical Editor SPi Global
Cover InTech Design team

First published March, 2018
Printed in Croatia
Legal deposit, Croatia: National and University Library in Zagreb

Additional hard copies can be obtained from orders@intechopen.com

Discussions of Unusual Topics in Fibromyalgia, Edited by William S. Wilke
p. cm.
Print ISBN 978-953-51-3899-0
Online ISBN 978-953-51-3900-3

For EU product safety concerns:
IN TECH d.o.o., Prolaz Marije Krucifikse Kozulić 3, 51000 Rijeka, Croatia, info@intechopen.com or visit our website at intechopen.com.

Meet the editor

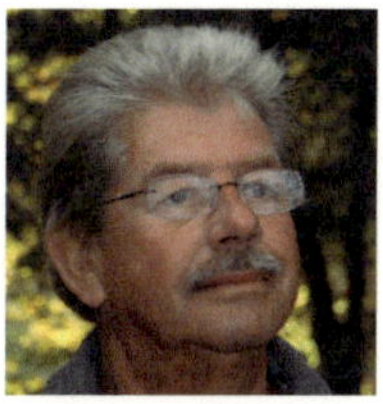

William S. Wilke received his Bachelor of Science degree from the University of Notre Dame and Doctor of Medicine degree from the Medical College of Wisconsin in 1971. He completed medical internship and residency at the Akron City Hospital. He completed rheumatology training and remained at the Cleveland Clinic Foundation (CCF) for 37 years, retiring in April 2011. He was working as a consultant/strategic advisor at the Crescendo Bioscience from 2012 to 2015. During his career at CCF, he was a chairman of the Medical Grand Rounds Committee and the Pharmacy and Therapeutics Committee, and the Head of Subspecialty Clinics from 1981 to 1995. From 1990 to 2011 (till retirement), he was an associate editor of the *Cleveland Clinic Journal of Medicine*. His outside activities included "Meet the Professor" as an expert in rheumatoid arthritis at the American College of Rheumatology Annual Meetings, 1991–1993, and he participated as a member of the United States Pharmacopeia General Committee, 1995–2000. Currently, he is the author of 132 various publications. He was the editor of the *Methotrexate Therapy in Rheumatic Disease*, Marcel Dekker Inc., 1989, and *New Insights into Fibromyalgia*, InTech, 2011. He was the author of *The Cleveland Clinic Guide to Fibromyalgia*, Kaplan Publishing, 2010.

Contents

Preface

I began my career in rheumatology in 1971. As an intern, I took over the rheumatology clinic on Wednesday mornings for indigent patients staffed by an intelligent, recently graduated rheumatologist. He knew all the latest about rheumatic diseases. In hindsight, it was not much.

In those days, we had an anemic treatment arsenal for most rheumatic diseases, including rheumatoid arthritis (RA) that, in fact, barely worked. Antimalarials, parenteral gold, corticosteroids, d-penicillamine, and the relatively new prostaglandin inhibitors such as ibuprofen were included among them [1]. The science of RA was also relatively primitive [2]. We knew that RA was an inflammatory disease, but immunology was in its infancy and consisted chiefly of T cells, B cells, serum complement, and a few circulating inflammatory proteins, one of which was associated with malignancy and caused wasting called cachectin, later named tumor necrosis factor-alpha.

Even more so for fibromyalgia syndrome (FMS), it was then known as fibrositis. Although a great many etiopathologic hypotheses existed, a "functional condition" was largely considered; that is, function was subjectively impaired, but no pathophysiologic abnormalities were evident [3]. Most local practitioners considered it as imaginary, prescribed "a sedative" or an opiate, and sent the patient away without follow-up [4].

Today, we have made fantastic strides in both understanding the pathophysiology and treating RA. We have identified various biochemical players in what we now know to be an extensive, redundant inflammatory cascade and blocked their activity. Remission or near-remission is now an achievable outcome [5].

Alternatively, although we understand some of the factors that play an etiopathologic role in FMS such as depression, anxiety, helplessness, disordered sleep, and poor physical conditioning, the biochemistry underlying and connecting these factors remains mysterious [6]. And unfortunately, even when we therapeutically manipulate a few mechanistic factors that we do understand such as serotonin or norepinephrine, the response is very limited [7].

Back in the early 1970s, most RA experts were opposed to the use of antineoplastic drugs or a combination of agents to improve inflammation in rheumatoid arthritis [8]. From my perspective, a rheumatology fellow who was being taught by Art Schebrel to use methotrexate and other cytotoxic agents in 1974 to treat various rheumatic diseases, I learned through contemporary literature, as well as angry calls and letters that the rheumatology community viewed this kind of treatment metaphorically as "A bull looking for a china shop." Anticipated unacceptably, high toxicity was the major issue [9]. Fortunately, those dire prophecies failed to materialize.

In retrospect, maybe the rheumatology community should have been a little more intellectually curious about new therapies for RA and novel etiopathogenic hypotheses. They also should have allowed themselves to be more skeptical about the results of contemporary treatment, the very modest outcomes associated with prevailing therapies, and the flawed etiopathogenic hypotheses. Had attitudes been a little more opened-minded, the treatment outcomes of RA and its science might have progressed more rapidly.

Our understanding of FMS pathogenesis and treatment remains relatively rudimentary compared to that of RA. So, it is in our and our patients' best interest to adopt those attitudes that were largely missing in understanding RA in 1970. We must remain open-minded manifested as curiosity a skepticism if the science of FMS and its treatment for FMS and its science is to progress. To that end, this book is useful.

Skepticism is the prominent intellectual attitude adopted in the first chapter. Because FMS is classified among autoimmune diseases and because most of the signs and symptoms including pain and fatigue are due to inflammatory autoimmune mechanisms, it might follow that the signs and symptoms of FMS are also due to inflammation. While it is true that inflammatory cytokines have been reported to be elevated in FMS in a few studies, the serologic concentrations in FMS are trivial compared to levels in active RA. It has also been shown that treatment with agents that nonspecifically lower serum cytokine concentrations do not improve signs and/or symptoms in FMS. Finally, primary depression, sleep disturbance, and other core FMS symptoms have been reported to be associated with similar low-level cytokine elevation that has been suggesting multifactorial etiology for any cytokine elevation in FMS.

In the second chapter, which is an exercise in curiosity, the authors present plausible hypotheses and provide preliminary data to show that oxidative stress plays at least a partial role in FMS etiopathogenesis.Dysfunction of both the endocrine and autonomic nervous systems is common in FMS, the etiology of which can be CNS damage from oxidation by free radicals. They invoke mitochondrial dysfunction as a primary explanation for this damage and show that antioxidants such as CoQ10 improve signs and symptoms associated with this damage. A curious attitude concludes that this concept begs further elucidation.

Chapter 3 should appeal to the skeptics. Western theories of treatment development are often reductionist, that is, discover the occult biological mechanisms underlying signs and symptoms, modify them, and expect reciprocal change. The skeptic might ask, "Why make it so difficult?" For instance, helplessness worsens the pain of FMS. Education reduces helplessness. Simple. Sleep is disrupted in FMS. Sleep hygiene is taught. Simple. The third chapter examines the studies that have shown empirical benefit from these practical interventions.

The fourth chapter appeals primarily to intellectual curiosity. The biological effects of substances that are "natural" can be mild-to-profound, beneficial, or not so much. Consider, for example, acetylsalicylic acid, on the positive side, and arsenic as an alternative. The authors provide well-referenced discussions of various natural products, efficacy trials, and clear descriptions of the beneficial effects and toxicities. They also address the mechanisms of action in the context of presumed FMS pathophysiology. We should expect that as these natural products are refined, just as digitalis leaf yielded a safer and more effective digoxin, new FMS medicines should emerge.

The last chapter invokes both skepticism and curiosity; skepticism is about the validity of outcome measures for some autoimmune diseases, in which pain and fatigue are the primary symptoms, and curiosity is about the phenotypic alterations by comorbid FMS. What does such a modification do to diagnostic criteria and measures of disease activity? As it turns out, when FMS is comorbid, the validity of outcome measures in the primary disease is modified, and diagnostic phenotypic changes are considerable. This is particularly true of indices that consist of subjective, patient-only-report measures. The resulting diagnostic and treatment considerations are discussed.

The science and treatment of FMS, when compared to that of RA, have much catching up to do. This little book about unusual FMS topics is a step in the right direction.

William S. Wilke MD,
Senior Staff Physician
Rheumatology Department, Orthopedic and Rheumatology Institute (retired)
Cleveland Clinic, Cleveland, OH, USA

References

[1] Schmid FR, Tesar JT, Rosen JS, et al. Rheumatoid arthritis. Postgraduate Medicine. 1971;**50**:143-149.

[2] Abruzzo JL. Rheumatoid arthritis: reflections on etiology and pathogenesis. Archives of Physical Medicine and Rehabilitation. 1971;**52**:30-38.

[3] Glyn JH. Rheumatic pains: some concepts and hypotheses. Proceedings of the Royal Society of Medicine. 1971;**64**:22-28.

[4] Kraft GH, Johnson EW, Laban MM. The fibrositis syndrome. Archives of Physical Medicine and Rehabilitation. 1968;**49**:155-162.

[5] Ruderman EM. Treating to target in rheumatoid arthritis – challenges and opportunities. Bulletin Hospital for Joint Diseases. 2013;**71**:214-217.

[6] Gracely RH, Schweinhardt P. Key mechanisms mediating fibromyalgia. Clinical and Experimental Rheumatology. 2015;**33**(Suppl. 88):S2-S6.

[7] Hauser W, Bernardy K, Uceyler N, Sommer C. Treatment of fibromyalgia syndrome with antidepressants. A meta-analysis. JAMA. 2009;**301**:198-209.

[8] Goldman JA, Hess EV. Treatment of rheumatoid arthritis-1970. Bulletin on the Rheumatic Diseases. 1970;**21**:609-612.

[9] Black RL, O'Brien WM, VanScot El, et al. Methotrexate therapy in psoriatic arthritis: double blind study on 21 patients. JAMA. 1964;**189**:743-747.

Chapter 1

Introductory Chapter: A Challenge to the Concept that Inflammation Plays a Prominent Pathogenic Role in Fibromyalgia

William S. Wilke

Additional information is available at the end of the chapter

http://dx.doi.org/10.5772/intechopen.72936

1. Introduction

Among the chapters in this monograph are those that examine the treatment of fibromyalgia syndrome (FMS) using nonpharmacologic natural products and other relatively novel agents [1–3]. Although the modes of therapy described are diverse, a role for disordered immune mechanisms is implicit in each of the three chapters. These include reference to sulfur springs considered to inhibit interleukin-2 and interferon-gamma [1], introductory explanations of FMS pathogenesis that invokes inflammatory dysfunction [2], and mention of inflammatory cytokine production associated with autonomic nervous system dysfunction-stimulated microglial and astrocyte cell activation [3]. The discussion in the fourth chapter about the impact of FMS on the evaluation of inflammatory diseases assumes the opposite that clinically significant inflammation is not a feature of FMS [4].

2. Case (should have been previously) closed

Face validity favoring a major pathogenic role for cytokine-mediated inflammation in FMS has been addressed in the past. Although initial reports of intermuscular fibrous tissue inflammation by Stockman led Gowers to name the condition "fibrositis," [5, 6], contemporary light and magnetic resonance imaging histological reports showed no evidence for peripheral muscle inflammation [7, 8]. These data should have closed the book on inflammation as a prominent etiopathogenic mechanism in FMS. Then along came inflammatory mediators.

In some contemporary reviews of FMS pathogenesis, inflammation is referenced in passing, as it is in these three chapters [9]. Whether this is done for "completeness," after all, FMS is often misclassified as a "connective tissue disease" (a misnomer), most of which are inflammatory in nature, or that such reference adds a sort of "scientific patina" to the discussion is unclear.

This review examines the validity of the concept that cytokine- and chemokine-driven inflammation is relevant to the pathogenesis of FMS.

3. Background

At least three observations have been used to provide circumstantial or hypothesis-generating evidence to advance a role for inflammatory pathogenesis:

1. The symptoms and signs of "sickness behavior" observed in FMS can be experimentally induced by inflammatory cytokines [10].
2. Similar alteration of the hypothalamic–pituitary axis and autonomic nervous system observed in FMS has been etiopathogenically linked to elevated inflammatory cytokines, including interleukin-1 (IL-1), in a variety of clinical settings other than FMS [11–14].
3. Symptoms of disordered sleep, hyperalgesia, and cognitive dysfunction much like FMS were observed when patients with renal cell carcinoma were treated with interleukin-2 lymphokine-activated killer (IL-2 LAK) cell therapy and when chronic hepatitis patients were treated with interferon alpha [15].

4. Experimental evidence for cytokine/chemokine pathogenesis

1. Previous inconsistent reports have demonstrated that C-reactive protein (CRP) can be marginally higher in FMS subjects than in parallel healthy controls [16]. In this analysis, however, serum inflammatory cytokines were not higher than in healthy controls.
2. Inconsistent elevation of a variety of serum cytokines has, however, been observed in some studies [16–24]. In a meta-analysis of 25 FMS studies, 1255 FMS, and 800 healthy controls (HC), interleukin-1 receptor antagonist (IL-1ra), interleukin-6 (IL-6), and interleukin-8 (IL-8) were the most likely inflammatory cytokines to be elevated [25].

Three integrated reviews, although acknowledging discrepancies in the literature, attempted to associate cytokine abnormalities with core FMS symptoms [26–28]. The first concluded, "There are discrepant findings related to whether pro-inflammatory and anti-inflammatory cytokines are elevated or reduced in persons with FMS and whether they correlate with core symptoms." [26]. The second [27] critiqued one of the more persuasive analysis, "….. may have cytokine driven abnormalities to explain their pain…IL-1ra and IL-6 were significantly higher after stimulating PBMC of FMS patients compared to controls [29]." The results of this study were not corroborated in a second study [24].

The third review of 12 separate analyses reported increased inflammatory cytokines IL-1ra, IL-6, and IL-8, and anti-inflammatory interleukin-10 (IL-10) or low anti-inflammatory interleukin-4 (IL-4) and IL-10 [24]. Among the inflammatory chemokines also linked to signs and symptoms, monocyte chemoattractant protein-1 (MCP-1), eotaxin among others, were elevated.

Two potentially innovative separate controlled analyses described cytokine and chemokine concentrations in the supernatant after mitogen stimulation of cultured monocytes, using a logistical regression model to achieve statistically determined weighting for each chemokine and cytokine, and offered this score as diagnostic test for FMS [30, 31]. Of interest, the inflammatory cytokines and chemokines including IL-6 were lower in concentration compared to healthy controls or individuals with autoimmune disease. These findings suggest increased damping control of inflammation in FMS. The authors of both these studies, however, failed to determine the prevalence of depression or analyze its potential effects on cytokine concentrations.

Among the most novel analyses was a report of elevation of intrathecal IL-8 derived from glia cells supporting the hypothesis that FMS symptoms might be mediated by glial cell activation through sympathetic nervous system mechanisms [32].

In summary, in individuals with FMS, peripheral blood IL-6, IL-1ra, and IL-8 concentrations may be a bit higher and IL-4 and IL-10 lower, and IL-8 may be relatively higher in the cerebral spinal fluid than in healthy controls. Inflammatory chemokines may also be higher than in healthy control patients.

5. Depression and inflammation

Depression and FMS are very often comorbid and show a bidirectional association [19, 33–38]. The prevalence of depression in FMS has been estimated to range from 20 to 80% in a detailed review [39]. Furthermore, the severity of comorbid depression correlates with FMS severity measures [40–42]. We have reported that depression, with a 73% prevalence, correlated better with core FMS symptoms than did any other variable in a cohort of 305 FMS patients [43].

As in FMS, similar mild elevation of CRP and inflammatory cytokines and chemokines have been demonstrated in depressed individuals in controlled analyses [44–53]. Many primary analyses of FMS inflammation [15, 30, 31, 54–56] and reviews [23, 28], however, failed to control for depression. This is an unfortunate omission.

Maes and colleagues evaluated the serum concentrations of inflammatory cytokines in relationship to depression among 21 FMS patients compared to 33 healthy controls [57].

Serum soluble gp130, an important inflammatory cytokine signal transducer, and a soluble interleukin-6 receptor, Il-1 ra, were significantly higher in FMS patients with a Hamilton Depression Rating Scale score >16 than in FMS patients with scores of 16 or lower or in healthy controls. In the opinion of the Menzies' integrated review, which included the Maes analysis, higher inflammatory cytokines in FMS, including IL6, were related to the degree of depression, although inconsistencies were common [26].

Of interest, higher body mass index partially explained cytokine differences as has been shown in depression [18, 52]. Therefore, inflammation in FMS, measured as higher serum concentrations of cytokines and chemokines, is multifactorial and not necessarily due solely to FMS pathophysiology.

Serum inflammatory cytokine concentrations correlate with the degree of depression and fall with effective treatment of depression [58]. Not surprisingly, inflammatory cytokine concentrations have also been shown to correlate with pain symptoms in primary depression alone [59].

This phenomenon even occurs when the treatment is nonpharmacological, suggesting an intrinsic etiopathophysiologic relationship of inflammatory cytokines with depression [46]. This analysis also demonstrated that despite a significant fall of cytokine concentration from baseline, the CRP was not significantly lower.

In summary, these two analyses demonstrate a pain symptom signature integral to depression and that cytokines, while slightly higher in depression than in healthy controls, are in fact trivial with respect to overall inflammation measured as CRP.

6. Different process mechanisms: RA versus FMS/depression

6.1. RA

In rheumatoid arthritis (RA) comorbid FMS is associated with disproportionately higher values for the subjective components, patient global assessment (PtGA), and tender joint count (TJC), which in turn inflate the disease activity score (DAS). This phenomenon is largely mediated by higher patient assessed pain, fatigue, and especially poor mood, and variables that define the criterion, distress, and the etiopathogenesis of FMS [60–64]. As a potential explanation, depression alone can disproportionately increase pain sensitivity, the tender joint count (TJC), and a patient's sense of wellbeing, such as PtGA in RA [19, 65]. Higher subjective signs and symptoms then inflate the DAS. It is important to note that concomitant FMS and depression in RA are not associated with obvious, clinically significant increases of CRP or erythrocyte sedimentation rate [42, 62, 65].

Differential response to the treatment of the so-called subjective versus objective variables is a hallmark of comorbid FMS and/or depression in RA. In a prospective analysis of 668 RA patients, 18% with comorbid FMS had higher DAS and Health Assessment Disability Index at baseline compared to patients without FMS [66]. The TJC and PtGA were significantly higher, but the objective factors, ESR, and swollen joint count (SJC) were significantly lower in patients with FMS compared to patients with RA alone. Achievement of low disease activity and remission were significantly less likely in the comorbid FMS cohort. Others have confirmed these observations [67].

A very instructive, early, placebo-controlled trial showed that the pain of FMS did not respond to the treatment with prednisone 15 mg/day [68]. So too, unlike dose-related reduction of objective signs in RA such as the swollen joint count (SJC) and CRP, FMS-related inflated subjective signs and symptoms are resistant to aggressive anti-immune, anti-inflammatory

RA treatment [69–71]. In fact, a treatment response resulting in remission in RA comorbid with FMS should not be expected because the higher, poorly responsive PtGA and TJC are not due to RA biological disease activity, but in fact to poorly responsive noninflammatory FMS central pain mechanisms [69].

7. Differential magnitude of inflammatory response

Mean CRP values, although reported elevated in some FMS populations compared to control populations, are still within the range of normal CRP [72]. Given this observation, it is both instructive and necessary to consider whether cytokines follow this same pattern.

7.1. Rewrite cytokine section

In RA, serum concentrations of IL-6 measured by enzyme immunoassay (ELISA) [73] in >900 patients demonstrated mean ~ 43 pg/ml, for all, and ~54–84 pg/ml for those with active disease [55]. In another population of 66 RA patients, using a similar assay, IL-6 levels declined to 22.5 pg/ml in low disease activity [74].

Contrast these serum levels with serum levels in depression and FMS. Using a different more sensitive ELISA assay, Grosse reported mean IL-6 serum concentration of 1.17 ± 2.59 for 214 patients with major depression disorder (MDD) and 0.66 ± 1.94 for healthy controls (HC) [50]. In another analysis of 64 MDD patients and 80 healthy controls, IL-6 levels were reported statistically higher in depression than in controls, 1.39 ± 0.35 versus 0.45 ± 0.28 pg/ml using yet another ELISA [47].

These same comparatively low serum levels were reported in FMS, with IL-6 in the range of 16 pg/ml in FMS and 1 pg/ml in healthy controls using yet another ELISA assay [75]. Although higher than HCs, the levels are very low when compared to those in RA.

This discussion apparently shows that inflammatory cytokines, even when relatively elevated in FMS, are much lower than in mildly active RA. If this is true, then the elevations in FMS may not be sufficiently high to initiate clinical signs or symptoms. Unfortunately, as can be seen, diverse assays that produce diverse serum and cellular concentrations and the lack of control for diurnal variation make precise comparisons between diseases difficult.

Fortunately, two papers do allow comparison. The authors of both studies used very similar ELISA methods. In 16 RA patients with varying disease activity, overnight IL-6 values ranged from a mean of ~40 pg/ml at 11 PM to a peak of ~60 at 8 AM with large individual variations [76].

In FMS, although the mean values for IL-6 were statistically significantly higher in FMS patients than in healthy controls at night (2.94 versus 2.14 pg/ml), these serum concentrations were at least 10 times lower in FMS than in RA [56]. Are these meager elevations of IL-6, ~0.80 pg/ml in FMS compared to HCs, sufficiently high enough to explain clinical differences?

Let us postulate that mildly elevated cytokines in the CNS such as IL-6 and IL-8 [32] produced by microglial and/or astrocyte cells are sufficient to interfere with processing and produce centrally mediated pain. We are still left with the lack of clinical response to moderate daily prednisone and even more aggressive antirheumatic, anti-inflammatory treatments which have been shown to reduce inflammation due to cytokines [67, 68, 71, 77].

There is little question that FMS does associate with mild cytokine change, such as reduced diurnal variation of IL-6 compared to healthy individuals [56]. Forensic objectivity, however, would seem to indicate that the described modest changes in inflammatory mediators, whether primary or secondary, do not seem sufficient to be responsible for clinically relevant FMS symptoms. Furthermore, in some very legitimate contemporary hypotheses of FMS etiopathogenesis, there is no role for chronic cytokine-mediated processes [78, 79].

8. Conclusions

The key points from this discussion are:

1. Although a minority of studies found CRP elevated in FMS compared to healthy controls, the mean high value was still within the normal range.
2. Depression, which is very often comorbid with FMS, was not well controlled in many cytokine/chemokine analyses. When it was, it was shown to significantly contribute to higher cytokine values.
3. Fibromyalgia symptoms, whether as the primary diagnosis or as comorbid in RA, do not respond to anti-inflammatory, anti-immune therapy.
4. Both stimulated and unstimulated cytokine and chemokine studies have employed a variety of methods of measurements that make cytokine levels difficult to analyze between diseases. A few comparisons have shown relatively trivial values in FMS compared to proven inflammatory disease such as RA.

Author details

William S. Wilke

Address all correspondence to: wswilkemd@gmail.com

Rheumatology Department, Clinic Orthopedic and Rheumatology Institute, Cleveland, OH, USA

References

[1] Kocak FA, Kurt EE. Nonpharmacologic Treatment of Fibromyalgia. InTech

[2] Brito RG, Santos PL, Olivera MA, et al. Natural Products as Promising Pharmacological Tools for the Management of Fibromyalgia Symptoms: A Review. InTech

[3] Miranda-Diaz AG, Odriguez-Lara SQ. The Role of Oxidants/Antioxidants, Mitochondrial Dysfunction, Autophagy in Fibromyalgia. InTech

[4] Wilke WS. Recognize Comorbid Fibromyalgia Syndrome in Order to Better Evaluate Rheumatic Diseases. InTech

[5] Stockman R. The causes, pathology and treatment of chronic rheumatism. Edinburgh Medical School. 1904;**15**:107-116

[6] Gowers WR. Lumbago. Its lessons and analogues. British Medical Journal. 1904;**114**: 117-121

[7] Fassbender HG, Wegner K. Morphologic and pathogenese des Weichteil rheumatismmus. Zeitschrift Fur Rheumaforsh. 1973;**32**:355-374

[8] Yunus MB, Kalyan-Raman UP, Masi AT, Aldag JC. Electron microscopic studies of muscle biopsy in primary fibromyalgia syndrome: A controlled and blinded study. The Journal of Rheumatology. 1989;**16**:97-101

[9] Arranz L-I, Canela M-A, Rafecas M. Fibromyalgia and nutrition, what do we know? Rheumatology International. 2010;**30**:1417-1427

[10] Dantzer R. Cytokine-induced sickness behavior a neuroimmune response to activation of innate immunity. European Journal of Pharmacology. 2004;**500**:399-411

[11] Dunne AJ. Cytokine activation of the HPA axis. Annals of the New York Academy of Sciences. 2000;**917**:608-617

[12] Wingenfeld K, Heim C, Schmidt I, et al. HPA axis reactivity and lymphocyte glucocorticoids sensitivity in fibromyalgia and pelvic pain. Psychosomatic Medicine. 2008;**242**:33-38

[13] Gur A, Oktayoglu P. Status of immune mediators in fibromyalgia. Current Pain Headache Reports. 2008;**12**:175-181

[14] Pillemer SR. The neuroscience and endocrinology of fibromyalgia. Arthritis & Rheumatism. 1997;**40**:1928-1939

[15] Wallace DJ, Margolin K, Waller P. Fibromyalgia and interleukin-2 therapy for malignancy. Annals of Internal Medicine. 1988;**106**:906

[16] Bazzichi L, Rossi A, Massimetti G, et al. Cytokine patterns in fibromyalgia and their correlation with clinical manifestation. Clinical and Experimental Rheumatology. 2007;**25**:225-230

[17] Hader N, Rimon D, Kinarty A, Lahat N. Altered interleukin-2 secretion in patients with primary fibromyalgia syndrome. Arthritis & Rheumatism. 1991;**34**:866-872

[18] Xiao Y, Haynes WL, Michalek JE, Russell IJ, et al. Elevated serum high-sensitivity C-reactive protein levels in fibromyalgia syndrome patients correlated with body mass index, interleukin-6, interleukin-8, erythrocyte sedimentation rate. Rheumatology International. May 2012;**33**(5):1259-1264. DOI: 10.1007/s00296-012-2538-6

[19] Toussaint LL, Vincent A, McSllister SJ, et al. Original experimental: A comparison of fibromyalgia symptoms in patients with Healthy versus depressive, low and reactive affect balance styles. Scandinavian Journal of Pain. 2014;**5**:161-166

[20] Tsiloni I, Russell IJ, Stewart JM, et al. Neuropeptides CRH, SP, HK-1, and inflammatory cytokines IL-6 and TNF are increased in serum of patients with fibromyalgia syndrome, implicating mast cells. Journal of Pharmacology and Experimental Therapeutics. 2016; **356**:664-672

[21] Gur A, Erdogan S, Nas K, et al. Regional cerebral blood flow and cytokines in young females with fibromyalgia. Clinical and Experimental Rheumatology. 2002;**20**:753-760

[22] Ortega E, Bote ME, Giraldo E, García JJ. Aquatic exercise improves the monocytes pro-and anti-inflammatorycytokine production balance in fibromyalgia patients. Scandivanian Journal of Medical Science and Sports. 2012;**22**:104-112

[23] Üçeyler N, Valenza R, Stock M, Schedel R, Sprotte G, Sommer C. Reduced levels of antiinflammatory cytokines in patients with chronic widespread pain. Arthritis & Rheumatism. 2006;**54**:2656-2664 [PubMed: 16871547]

[24] Kashipaz MRA, Swindon D, Todd I, et al. Normal production of inflammatory cytokines in chronic fatigue and fibromyalgia syndromes determined by intracellular cytokine staining in short-term cultured blood mononuclear cells. Clinical and Experimental Immunology. 2003;**132**:360-365

[25] Uceyler N, Hauser W, Sommer C. Systemic review with meta-analysis: Cytokines in fibromyalgia syndrome. BMC Musculoskeletal Disorders. 2011;**12**:245-260

[26] Menzies V, Lyon DE. Integrated review of the association of cytokines with fibromyalgia and fibromyalgia core symptoms. Biological Research for Nursing. 2010;**11**:387-394

[27] Staud R. Cytokine and immune system abnormalities in fibromyalgia and other central sensitivity syndromes. Current Rheumatology Review. 2015;**11**:109-115

[28] Rodriguez-Pinto I, Agmon-Levin N, Howard A, Shoenfeld Y. Fibromyalgia and cytokines. Immunology Letters. 2014;**161**:200-203

[29] Wallace DJ, Linker-Israeli M, Hallegua D, et al. Cytokines play an aetiopathogenetic role in fibromyalgia: A hypothesis and pilot study. Rheumatology. 2001;**40**:743-749

[30] Behm FG, Gavin IW, Karpenko O, et al. Unique immunologic patterns in fibromyalgia. BMC Clinical Pathology. 2012;**12**:25-32

[31] Wallace DJ, Gavin IG, Karpenko O, et al. Cytokine and chemokine profiles in fibromyalgia, rheumatoid arthritis and systemic lupus erythematosus: A potentially useful tool in differential diagnosis. Rheumatology International. 2015;**35**:991-996

[32] Kadetoff D, Lampa J, Westman M, et al. Evidence of central inflammation in fibromyalgia—Increased cerebrospinal fluid interleukin-8 levels. Neuroimmunology. 2012;**242**:33-38

[33] Krag NJ, Norregaard J, Larsen JK, Danneskiold-Samsoe B. A blinded controlled evaluation of anxiety and depressive symptoms in patients with fibromyalgia, as measured by standardized psychometric interview scales. Acta Psychiatrica Scandinavica. 1994;**89**:370-375

[34] Hudson JI, Hudson MS, Pliner LF, Goldenberg DL, Pope, HG Jr. Fibromyalgia and major affective disorder: A controlled phenomenology and family history study. American Journal of Psychiatry. 1985;**142**:441-446

[35] Hudson JI, Pope HG. Fibromyalgia and psychopathology: Is fibromyalgia a form of affective spectrum disorder? Journal of Rheumatology (suppl.). 1989;**19**:15-22

[36] Hudson JI, Goldenberg DL, Pope HG, Keck PE, Schlesinger L. Comorbidity of fibromyalgia with medical and psychiatric disorders. American Journal of Medicine. 1992; **92**:363-367

[37] Gruber AJ, Hudson JI, Pope HG. The management of treatment-resistant depression in disorders on the interface of psychiatry and medicine. Fibromyalgia, chronic fatigue syndrome, migraine, irritable bowel syndrome, a typical facial pain, and premenstrual dysphoric disorder. Psychiatry Clinics of North America. 1996;**19**:351-369

[38] Chang M-H, Hsu J-W, Huang K-I, et al. Bidirectional association between depression and fibromyalgia syndrome: A nationwide longitudinal study. Journal of Pain. Sep 2015;**16**(9):895-902. DOI: 10.1016/j.jpain.2015.06.004

[39] Fieta P, Manganelli P. Fibromyalgia and psychiatric disorders. Acta Biomedica. 2007;**78**:88-95

[40] Hawley DJ, Wolfe F. Depression is not more common in rheumatoid arthritis: A 10-year longitudinal study of 6153 patients with rheumatic disease. Journal of Rheumatology. 1993;**20**:2025-2031

[41] Arnold LM, Hudson JI, Keck PE, et al. Comorbidity of fibromyalgia and psychiatric disorders. Journal of Clinical Psychiatry. 2006;**67**:1219-1225

[42] Brown D, Mulvey M, Cordingley L, et al. The relationship between psychological distress and multiple tender points across the adult lifespan. Archives of Gerontology and Geriatrics. 2016;**63**:102-107

[43] Gota CE, Kauok S, Wilke WS. The impact of depressive and bipolar symptoms on socioeconomic status, core symptoms, function and severity of fibromyalgia. International Journal of Rheumatic Diseases. 2015;**20**(3):326-339

[44] Wium-Andersen MK, Orsted MD, Nielsen SF, Nordestgaard BG. Elevated C-reactive protein levels, psychological distress, and depression in 73131 individuals. JAMA Psychiatry. 2013;**70**:176-184

[45] Berk M, Wadee AA, Kruschke RH, O'neil-Kerr A. Acute phase proteins in major depression. Journal of Psychosomatic Research. 1997;**43**:529-534

[46] Dahl J, Ormstad H, HCD A, et al. The plasma levels of various cytokines are increased during ongoing depression and are reduced to normal levels after recovery. Psychoneuroendocrinology. 2014;**45**:77-86

[47] Fan N, Luo Y, Ou Y, He H. Altered serum levels of TNF-alpha, IL-6, and IL-18 in depressive disorder patients. Human Psychopharmacology Clinical and Experiment. 2017;**32**:e2588. https://doi.org/10.1002/hup.2588

[48] Goldsmith DR, Rapaport MH, Miller BJ. A meta-analysis of blood cytokine network alterations in psychiatric patients: Comparisons between schizophrenia, bipolar disorder and depression. Molecular Psychiatry. 2016;**21**(12):1696-1709

[49] Davami MH, Baharlou R, Vasmehjani AA, et al. Elevated IL-17 and TGF-β serum levels: A positive correlation between T-helper 17 cell-related pro-inflammatory responses with major depressive disorder. Basic and Clinical Neuroscience. 2015;**7**(2):137-142

[50] Grosse L, Ambree O, Jorgens S, et al. Cytokine levels in major depression are related to childhood trauma but not to recent stressors. Psychoneuroendocrinology. 2016; **73**:24-31

[51] Eyre HA, Air T, Pradham A, et al. A meta-analysis of chemokines in major depression. Progress in Neuro-psychopharmacology & Biological Psychiatrtry. 2016;**68**:1-8. DOI: 10.1016/j.pnpbp.2016.02006

[52] Howren B, Lamkin DM, Suls J. Associations of depression with C-reactive protein, IL-1, and IL-6: A meta analysis. Psychosomatic Medicine. 2009;**71**:171-186

[53] Dowlati Y, Hermann N, Swardfager W, et al. A meta-analysis of cytokines in major depression. Biological Psychiatry. 2010;**67**:446-457

[54] Zhang Z, Cherryholmes G, Mao A, et al. High plasma levels of MCP-1 and eotaxin provide evidence for an immunological basis of fibromyalgia. Experimental Biology and Medicine (Maywood). 2008;**233**:1171-1180

[55] Wang J, Platt A, Upmanyu R, et al. IL-6 pathway-driven investigation of response to IL-6 receptor inhibition in rheumatoid arthritis. BMJ Open. 2013;**3**:e003199. DOI: 10.1136/bmjopen-2013-003199

[56] Fatima G, Mahdi AA, Das SK, et al. Lack of circadian pattern of serum TNF-a and IL-6 in patients with fibromyalgia syndrome. Indian Journal of Clinical Biochemistry. 2012;**27**:(4)340-343 (October–December 2012)

[57] Maes M, Libbrect I, Van Hunsel F, et al. The immune-inflammatory pathophysiology of fibromyalgia: Increased serum soluble gp130, the common signal transducer protein of various neurotrophic cytokines. Psychoneuroendocrinology. 1999;**24**:371-383

[58] Hannestad J, DellaGioia N, Bloch M. The effect of antidepressant medication treatment on serum levels of inflammatory cytokines: A meta-analysis. Neuropsychopharmacology. 2011;**36**:2452-2459

[59] Bai Y-A, Chou W-F, Su T-P, et al. Pro-inflammatory cytokine associated with somatic and pain symptoms in depression. Journal of Affective Disorders. 2014;**155**:28-34

[60] Wolfe F, Clauw DJ, Fitzcharles MA, Goldenberg DL, Katz RS, Mease P, et al. The American College of Rheumatology preliminary diagnostic criteria for fibromyalgia and measurement of symptom severity. Arthritis Care Research. 2010;**62**:600-610

[61] Fifield J, Tennen H, Reisine S, McQuillan J. Depression and the long-term risk of pain, fatigue, and disability in patients with rheumatoid arthritis. Arthritis & Rheumatism. 1998;**41**:1851-1857

[62] Kapoor SR, Hider SJ, Brownfield A, et al. Fibromyalgia in patients with rheumatoid arthritis. Clinical and Experimental Rheumatology. 2011;**29**(Suppl. 69):S88-S91

[63] Wolfe F, Michaud K, Busch RE, et al. Polysymptomatic distress in patients with rheumatoid arthritis: Understanding disproportionate response and its spectrum. Arthritis Care Research (Hoboken). 2014;**66**(10):1465-1471

[64] Lee YC, Bingham CO III, Edwards RR, et al. Pain sensitization is associated with disease activity in rheumatoid arthritis patients: A cross-sectional study. Arthritis Care and Research. 2017; Accepted Article. DOI: 10.1002/acr.23266

[65] Matcham F, Ali S, Irving K, et al. Are depression and anxiety associated with disease activity in rheumatoid arthritis? A prospective study. BMC Musculoskeletal Disorder. 2016;**17**:155

[66] Kim H, Cui J, Frits M, et al. Fibromyalgia predicts two-year changes in functional status in rheumatoid arthritis patients. Arthritis Care Research. Dec 2017;**69**(12):1871-1877. Accepted Article'. DOI: 10.1002/acr.23216

[67] Duran J, Combe B, Niu J, et al. The effect on treatment response of fibromyalgic symptoms in early rheumatoid arthritis patients: Results from the ESPOIR cohort. Rheumatology. 2015;**54**:2166-2170

[68] Clark S, Tindall E, Bennett RM. A double blind crossover trial of prednisone versus placebo in the treatment of fibrositis. Journal of Rheumatology. 1985;**12**:980-983

[69] Lee YC, Cui J, Lu B, et al. Pain persists in DAS28 rheumatoid arthritis remission but not in ACR/EULAR remission: A longitudinal observational study. Arthritis Research & Therapy. 2011;**R13**:R83

[70] Lage-Hansen PR, Chrysidis S, Lage-Hansen M, et al. Concomorbid fibromyalgia in rheumatoid arthritis is associated with the more frequent use of biological therapy: Across-sectional study. Scandinavian Journal of Rheumatology. Jan 2016;**45**(1):45-48

[71] Altawil R, Saevarsdottir S, Wedren S, et al. Remaining pain in early rheumatoid arthritis patients treated with methotrexate. Arthritis Care Research. 2016;**68**:1061-1068

[72] Feinberg T, Sambamoorthi U, Lilly C, Innes KK. Potential mediators between fibromyalgia and C-reactive protein: Results from a Large U.S. Community Survey. BMC Musculoskeletal Disorders. 2017;**18**:294. DOI: 10.1186/s12891-017-1641-y

[73] Fraunberger P, Pfeiffer M, Cremer P. et al, Validation of an automated enzyme immunoassay for iInterleukin-6 for routine clinical use. Clinical Chemical and Laboratory Medicine. 1998;**36**:797-801

[74] Robak T, Gladalska A, Stepien H, et al. Serum levels of interleukin-6 type cytokines and soluble interleukin-6 receptor in patients with rheumatoid arthritis. Mediators Inflammation. 1998;**7**:347-353

[75] Hernandez ME, Becerril E, Perez M, et al. Proinflammatory cytokine levels in fibromyalgia patients are independent of body mass index. BMC Research Notes. 2010;**3**:156

[76] Perry MG, Kirwan JR, Jessop DS, Hunt LP. Overnight variations in cortisol, interleukin 6, tumour necrosis factor alpha and other cytokines in people with rheumatoid arthritis. Annals of the Rheumatic Diseases. 2009;**68**:63-68

[77] Vermeer M, Kuper HH, van der Bijl AE, et al. The provision al ACR/EULAR definition of remission in RA: A comment on the patient global assessment criterion. Rheumatology. 2012;**51**:1076-1080

[78] Gracely RH, Schweinhardt P. Key mechanisms mediating fibromyalgia. Clinical and Experimental Rheumatology. 2015;**33**(Suppl. 88):S3-S6

[79] Cagnie B, Coppieters I, Denecker S, et al. Central sensitization in fibromyalgia? A systematic review on structural and functional brain MRI. Seminars Arthritis Rheumatism. 2014;**44**:68-75

Chapter 2

The Role of Oxidants/Antioxidants, Mitochondrial Dysfunction, and Autophagy in Fibromyalgia

Alejandra Guillermina Miranda-Díaz and
Simón Quetzalcóatl Rodríguez-Lara

Additional information is available at the end of the chapter

http://dx.doi.org/10.5772/intechopen.70695

Abstract

Fibromyalgia (FM) is a syndrome that presents primarily in women and is characterized by generalized pain, muscle rigidity, poor quality of sleep, fatigue, cognitive dysfunction, anxiety, episodes of depression, overall sensitivity, and deterioration in the performance of day-to-day activities. In the pathophysiology of fibromyalgia neuroendocrine factors, anomalies of the autonomous nervous system, genetic characteristics, and environmental and psychosocial factors are implicated. Alterations to the cells of the central nervous system that are present in fibromyalgia are due to the toxic effects of free radicals by the high concentrations of polyunsaturated fatty acids of the membranes that are easily oxidized and the low level of protective antioxidant enzymes. In FM, defects are produced in any part of the cycle in the generation of adenosine-5′-triphosphate (ATP) by the mitochondria, which can alter energy production by the mitochondria and cause the characteristic symptoms of FM. The degradation of the mitochondria dependent on autophagy or mitophagy is an important process for maintaining the critical integrity of the mitochondria and limiting the production of reactive oxygen species (ROS). Therefore, the deregulation of autophagy and mitochondrial dysfunction could represent key aspects in the pathophysiology of FM. Management with antioxidants, vitamins, coenzyme Q10, and melatonin, in addition to the antidepressants and structural analogs of the gamma-aminobutyric acid, could modify the florid symptomatology that patients with FM have.

Keywords: fibromyalgia, oxidative stress, mitochondrial dysfunction, autophagy, antioxidants, antioxidant vitamins

1. Introduction

1.1. Fibromyalgia

Fibromyalgia (FM) is a syndrome characterized by generalized pain, muscle rigidity, poor quality of sleep, fatigue, cognitive dysfunction, anxiety, episodes of depression, overall sensitivity, and deterioration in the performance of day-to-day activities [1, 2]. The incidence of FM is higher in women than in men in all decades of life, and it generally appears between 30 and 35 years of age [3, 4]. The prevalence of FM increases with age, reaching a maximum peak around the seventh decade. Fibromyalgia affects about 5% of the population worldwide [5]. According to the classification of the American College of Rheumatology, the definition of FM encompasses two variables: (a) bilateral pain above and below the waist with centralized pain and (b) chronic generalized pain for 3 months with pain on palpation in at least 11 of 18 specific body sites (sensitive spots) [6]. In the presentation of FM alterations to the central and autonomous nervous system, and alterations to the neurotransmitters, hormones, the external immune system, psychiatric conditions, and stress factors are involved [7]. Along with pain there are frequent disturbances in sleep, fatigue, morning rigidity, a subjective sensation of the accumulation of bodily fluids, paresthesias of the extremities, depression, headache, dizziness, and intestinal disturbances, which cause a decrease in quality of life [8]. The current review describes the oxidative stress, mitochondrial alterations, autophagy, antioxidants, and alternatives to the pharmacological management of FM.

1.2. Etiology

The etiology and the pathophysiological mechanisms of FM are still unknown and continue to be a challenging clinical entity for researchers and clinicians [9]. Some studies suggest that the involvement of the hypothalamus-pituitary–adrenal axis and the autonomic nervous system in response to stress is present in patients who are vulnerable to suffering with FM or its symptoms [10]. Neuroendocrine factors, anomalies of the autonomic nervous system, genetic characteristics, environmental changes, psychosocial changes, and oxidative stress are involved in the pathophysiology of FM [11]. There is a high prevalence of FM among relatives of patients who also suffer from it, which is attributed to the combination of environmental and genetic factors [12]. Genetic studies suggest that the association with polymorphisms of the serotoninergic, dopaminergic, and catecholaminergic pathways found is implicated in the transmission and modulation of pain [11]. One theory of etiology suggests that infections are capable of activating inflammatory cytokines that could modify the central and peripheral perception of pain in FM. FM is characterized by chronic pain of unknown origin. Evidence suggests that sensitized neurons in the spinal cord of the dorsal horn are responsible for processing increased pain from peripheral nociceptive signals, glial activation, apparently by cytokines and excitatory amino acids that could play a role in the initiation and perpetuation of the pain due to acute or repetitive tissue injury [13]. Three FM subgroups have been described based on the predominant symptoms, depending on the following domains: psychosocial (depression/anxiety), cognitive (catastrophic/pain control), and neurobiology (sensitivity) [14]. The proportion of new patients with FM varies between

http://dx.doi.org/10.5772/intechopen.70695

10 and 20% in clinics for patients with rheumatic diseases, while in clinics not specialized for rheumatic illnesses the prevalence is >2.1–5.7% [15]. Amitriptyline is the most common prescription drug for the management of FM. Amitriptyline has the ability to influence the autonomic nervous system [16].

2. Oxidative stress

Oxygen is used by the eukaryotic cells for metabolic transformations and the production of energy by the mitochondria. Under physiologic conditions, there is a beneficial endogenous production of reactive oxygen species (ROS) and reactive nitrogen species (RNS) that interact as signaling molecules in multiple physiological mechanisms (**Figure 1**). The ROS have bactericide activity of the phagocytes, act in the transduction of signals, and in the regulation of cellular growth and the redox state of the cell, among other mechanisms [17]. When the ROS or RNS are produced in excess or are not eliminated by the antioxidants, the oxidative stress with the capacity to damage the macromolecules (carbohydrates, proteins, lipids, DNA, and organelles) is produced [18, 19]. In relation to FM, it is important to mention that the cells of the central nervous system are highly vulnerable to the toxic effects of free radicals when

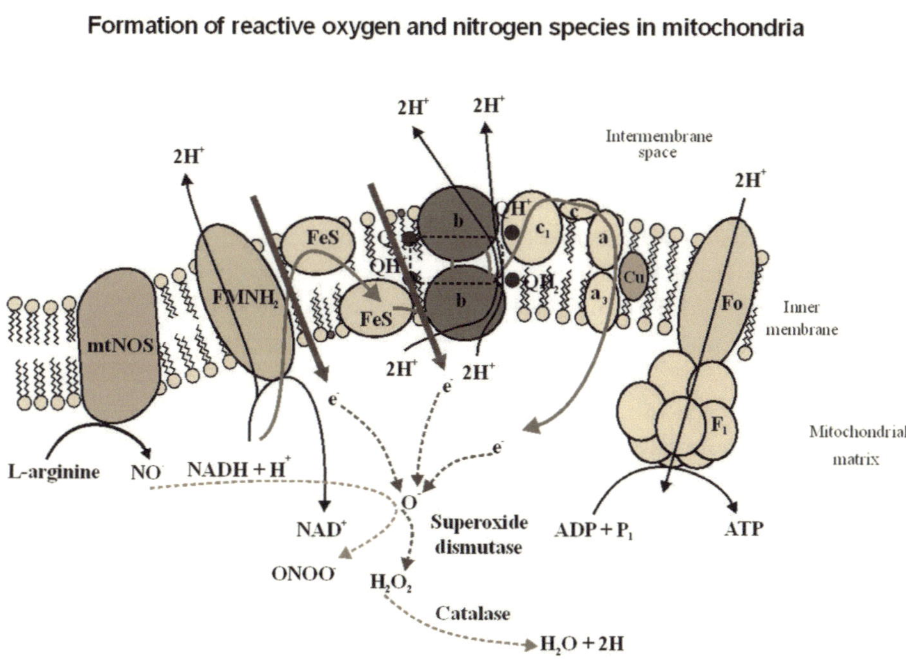

Figure 1. Formation of reactive oxygen and nitrogen species in mitochondria. The process is mediated by oxidative phosphorylation and the activity of the mitochondrial NO synthase: In physiological conditions, the production of ROS and RNS is reduced by multiple enzymatic scavengers that involved SOD, GPx, and catalase. When the mitochondria suffer an insult, the increase of the leakage of electrons to the matrix leads to an overload to the capacity of the enzymatic systems and leads to toxicity of the cell. Vectors of reactions and products. The physiological pathway for formation of oxidative stress. Leakage of electron to matrix. Pathophysiological pathway for formation of ROS and RNS.

compared to other organs in the body because they have a high index of oxidative metabolic activity and a low level of protector antioxidant enzymes, with an anatomical neuronal network that is vulnerable to interruption and high concentrations of polyunsaturated fatty acids of the membrane that are easily oxidized [20]. One of the primary enzyme sources of the superoxide anion (O^{2-}) is the xanthine oxidase. The purine nucleotides are degraded where the phosphate group is lost by the action of the 5′-nucleotidase. The adenosine is deaminated to inosine by the adenosine deaminase (ADA). The inosine is hydrolyzed to produce the purine base hypoxanthine, which is subsequently oxidized to xanthine and later to uric acid by the xanthine oxidase. The xanthine oxidase is an important enzyme that contains iron and molybdenum. The enzyme exists primarily in the form of xanthine dehydrogenase and can convert into xanthine oxidase through diverse conditions including proteolysis, homogenization, and the oxidation of sulfhydryl [21]. Oxidative stress appears to be involved in the severity of symptoms in FM; thus, the antioxidant therapy should be investigated as a possible alternative to adjunct management of FM. Blockage of the production of ROS by the mitochondria offers a new therapeutic strategy to diminish the symptoms of FM and other inflammatory states.

2.1. Lipoperoxides in fibromyalgia

The overproduction of ROS favors lipid peroxidation (LPO) that leads to the oxidative destruction of the polyunsaturated fatty acids, components of the cellular membranes, and favors the production of cytotoxic metabolites and aldehyde reactives [malondialdehyde (MDA) and 4-hydroxynonenal (HNE)] [22]. The MDA and HNE produced in relatively large quantities have an important capacity for diffusion from their site of origin and attack distant objects to form covalent bonds with diverse molecules [23]. Measuring MDA is one popular method in the search for LPO in bodily fluids or cell lysates. In one study reported in 2011, the authors found increased levels of LPO in mononuclear cells associated with the plasma levels of LPO and clinical symptoms of FM, within the pathophysiology of FM [24]. Research in LPO is highly important since the deleterious effects of oxidative stress could be prevented through control of the underlying pathology and the administration of antioxidants or free radical scavengers.

2.2. Nitric oxide in fibromyalgia

The production of nitric oxide (NO) occurs from the L-arginine by the nitric oxide synthase (NOS) (**Figure 2**). The NOS has four isoforms: neuronal (nNOS), inducible (iNOS), endothelial (eNOS), and mitochondrial (mtNOS) [25]. The NO is implicated in physiological processes like: vasodilation, modulation of nociception, immune function, neurotransmission, and excitation-contraction coupling [26]. The NO is considered an atypical neurotransmitter and a second messenger in the nervous system [27] or as a hormone [28]. The majority of the effects of NO are mediated through the activation of the guanylate-cyclase enzyme that produces cyclic guanosine-3,5-monophosphate (cGMP) [29]. The NO has pro-nociceptor properties in the neural crest and in the dorsal root ganglia that positively regulate as a result of cutaneous or visceral inflammation and by the peripheral lesions of the fibers. This effect could be

http://dx.doi.org/10.5772/intechopen.70695

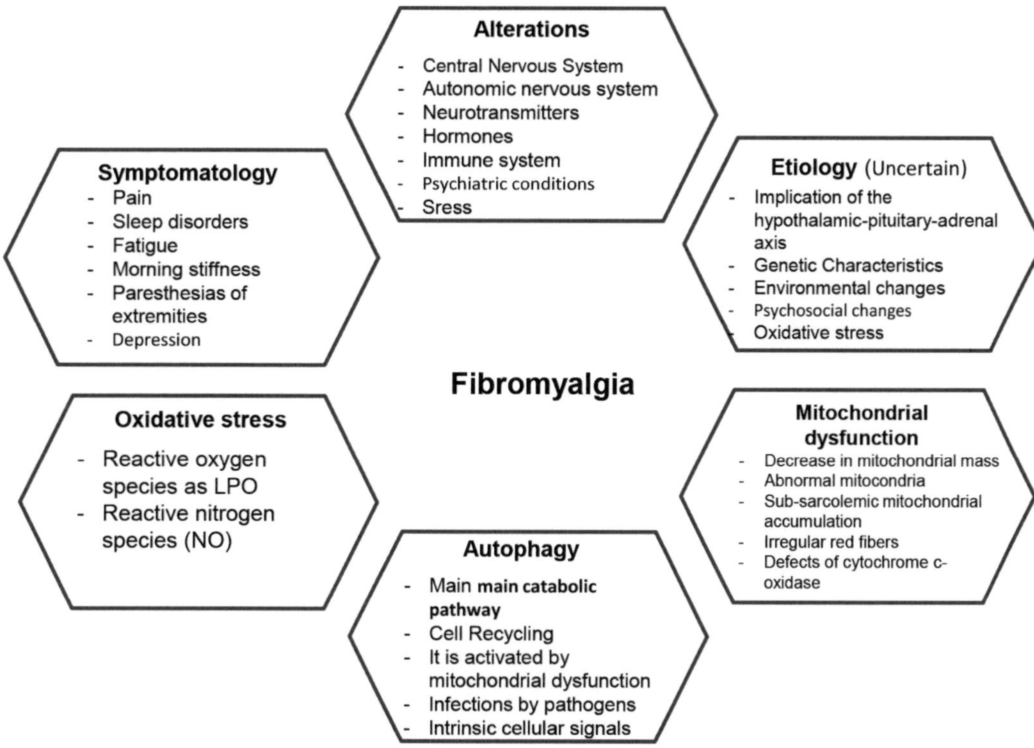

Figure 2. Mechanisms involved in the presentation of fibromyalgia. The alterations involved in the presentation of fibromyalgia. The etiology and symptomatology of the appearance of fibromyalgia and events may be the cause or consequence of having FM.

potentiated or inhibited by the NO donors [29]. In addition, a decrease in capillary volume of the blood vessels, structural disorganization of the capillary endothelium, and structural abnormalities of the mitochondria in histopathology studies of muscles have been reported in FM [30]. The structural damages can contribute to poor oxygen diffusion, less oxidative phosphorylation, and a decrease in the synthesis of ATP, which can increase oxidative stress and LPO of the membrane [31]. Abnormal microcirculation of the skin above sensitive spots in patients with FM has been reported with the use of the laser Doppler flowmetry technique [32]. The results support that local hypoxia and the possible decrease in concentrations of high-energy phosphate result in oxidative stress and LPO of the membrane. Therefore, abnormal microcirculation can be a result of the abnormal regulation of capillary blood flow [33].

3. Mitochondrial alterations in fibromyalgia

Mitochondrial myopathies are disturbances that are characterized by morphological anomalies of the mitochondria in muscles. Mitochondrial problems are found in the most common inherited metabolic illnesses. The patients who suffer from mitochondrial myopathies can present symptomatology characterized by muscle weakness, pain, fatigue, and exercise intolerance that progressively worsen over time, similar to what happens in patients with FM [34]. Defects in any part of the cycle in the generation of ATP by the mitochondria can alter mitochondrial energy production and cause symptoms [35]. Oxidative stress is implicated in the pathogenesis of FM, which indicates that mitochondrial dysfunction can be associated with FM [36]. In fact, a decrease in the quantity of mitochondrial mass and the coenzyme Q10 (CoQ10) in the production of mitochondrial ROS in mononuclear blood cells has been detected in patients who suffer from FM [37]. Reports of muscle biopsies from the trapezius muscle have shown inflammatory markers, abnormal mitochondria, accumulation of sub-sarcolemma mitochondria, higher incidence of irregular red fibers, and defects of the cytochrome-c oxidase (Complex IV of oxidative phosphorylation) [38]. In addition, the implication of mitochondrial oxidative stress in peripheral nociception described as a predominant symptom mediated by the inflammatory state in FM has been previously reported [39].

4. Autophagy

Autophagy is the process of cellular recycling that promotes energy efficiency through the generation of ATP and mediates damage control through the elimination of organelles and nonfunctional proteins, in regulating the degradation of cytosolic components by the liposomes [40]. Autophagy is the main catabolic pathway through which macromolecules and organelles of the eukaryotic cells are degraded and recycled. This pathway is activated under conditions of environmental stress and during the development of diverse pathologic situations. Autophagy plays an essential role in the cellular differentiation, development, and response to stress. It is activated during amino acid deprivation and is associated with neurodegenerative illnesses, cancer, pathogenic infections, and myopathies [41]. Autophagy can be induced by diverse causes: mitochondrial dysfunctions, infections of intracellular pathogens, and intrinsic cellular signals. Folded or damaged proteins, the organelles, and the intracellular pathogens are isolated by double membrane vesicles forming autophagosomes, which, on fusing with the lysosomes, convert into autolysosomes to be degraded [42]. Autophagy is an active process that plays the role of cleansing in maintaining the integrity of the intracellular organelles and proteins; however, autophagy is strongly induced by starvation, as in the case of cellular hypoxia, and is a key component in the adaptive response of the cells and organisms to the lack of nutrients, in order to promote cellular survival until the nutrients are made available once more [43]. Thirty-two different genes have been identified in relation to autophagy, obtained by genetic screening in yeasts. Many of these genes can be found in mold, plants, worms, flies, and in mammals, emphasizing, through phylogeny, the importance of the autophagy process in response to starvation [44]. Three types of autophagy that promote proteolytic degradation of the cytosolic components in lysosomes have been defined:

a. *Macroautophagy:* the cytoplasmic load is given to the lysosomes through a vesicle with a double-layered membrane called an autophagosome, which fuses with the lysosome to form the autolysosome. Macroautophagy is capable of engulfing large structures through selective and nonselective mechanisms.

http://dx.doi.org/10.5772/intechopen.70695

b. *Microautophagy:* the cytosolic components are absorbed directly by the lysosome through engulfment by the lysosomal membrane. In microautophagy, large structures can also be ingested through selective and nonselective mechanisms.

c. *Chaperone-mediated autophagy:* targeted proteins are translocated through the lysosomal membrane forming a complex with protein chaperones (i.e., Hsc-70) that are recognized by the membrane protein 2A associated with the lysosomes of the lysosomal membrane, causing unfolding and degradation [45].

The autophagy mechanism begins with an isolation membrane (phagophore), probably derived from the lipid bilayer originating in the endoplasmic reticulum (ER), and/or through the Golgi apparatus and endosomes [46]. The phagophore expands to engulf intracellular components, isolating protein aggregates, organelles and ribosomes, and forming an autophagosome with a double membrane. The autophagosome matures through fusion with the lysosome, promoting the degradation of the autophagosome content by acidic lysosome proteases. The lysosomal permeases and transporters export amino acids and by-products of degradation to the cytoplasm, where they can be reused for the construction of macromolecules and for metabolism [47]. Selective degradation of the mitochondria mediated by autophagy is called mitophagy [48]. It seems the absence of functional mitochondria produced by metabolic deregulation and autophagy obligates the muscle cells to gain energy without the participation of the Krebs cycle, in comparison to intact mitochondria. The mitochondrial degradation dependent on autophagy or mitophagy is an important process to maintain the critical integrity of the mitochondria and to limit the production of ROS [49]. The deregulation of autophagy and mitochondrial dysfunction could represent key aspects in the pathophysiology of FM [50]. The authors demonstrate that CoQ deficient fibroblasts exhibit increased levels of lysosomal markers (beta-galactosidase, cathepsin, LC3, and Lyso Tracker), and enhanced expression of autophagic genes at both transcriptional and translational levels, indicating the presence of autophagy [51]. CoQ10 deficiency apparently induces autophagy activation in mononuclear blood cells (BMCs) of FM patients by finding increased levels of acid vacuoles in BMCs identified by Lysotracker fluorescence and flow cytometry analysis. The authors suggest restoring mitochondrial functionality with CoQ10 supplementation as demonstrated in *in vitro* studies with decreased lysosomal activity following treatment with CoQ10 [52]. Autophagy is an attractive, strategic target for investigation of bodily fluids or muscle biopsies in patients who suffer FM (**Figure 2**).

5. Managing fibromyalgia

Treatment for FM is a challenge and often requires nonpharmacological and pharmacological treatment [53]. The dietary habits of FM patients are important, and diverse studies have demonstrated improvement of symptoms with the ingestion of healthy, balanced diets [54]. However, the heterogeneity of symptoms that presents in FM deserves individualized treatment. Therapy should include physiotherapy, psychotherapy, pharmacotherapy, and educate the patient on the pathology of FM [55].

5.1. Amitriptyline in fibromyalgia

Amitriptyline is a tricyclic antidepressant known to inhibit the reuptake of serotonin and norepinephrine, and it has been used for a long period of time in the management of neuropathic pain and FM [56]. Amitriptyline is the pharmacological treatment with the most solid evidence in FM management, although exhaustive follow-up for secondary effects is recommended [57]. The administration of the medication is recommended for short periods to control pain. It was previously reported that the administration of 50 mg/day of amitriptyline at bedtime, for 9 weeks, in patients with FM, significantly improved pain, muscle rigidity, and sleep, compared to patients treated with placebo [58]. In another study, 62 patients with FM received 25 mg/day of amitriptyline at bedtime with an additional 500 mg of naproxen x2 daily, or a placebo for 6 weeks. Those who received amitriptyline had significant improvements in pain, sleep disturbances, and fatigue on waking, compared to those who received placebo. The authors did not find significant differences in improvement of pain among patients who only received amitriptyline or amitriptyline with naproxen [59]. The guidelines of the European League Against Rheumatism (EULAR) suggest that the management of FM with low doses of amitriptyline of 25 mg/day improves pain, sleep, and fatigue at 6–8 weeks without finding evidence that the use of 50 mg/day was superior [60]. However, the toxicity induced by amitriptyline implies the early activation of the mitofagia that subsequently changes to apoptosis. Amitriptyline induces mitochondrial dysfunction and oxidative stress in HepG2 cells. Amitriptyline specifically inhibits mitochondrial complex III activity that is associated with decreased mitochondrial membrane potential ($\Delta\Psi m$) and increased ROS production. Transmission electron microscopy studies revealed structurally abnormal mitochondria that were engulfed by double membrane structures resembling autophagosomes. Pharmacological or genetic inhibition of autophagy exacerbated the deleterious effects of amitriptyline on hepatoma cells and leads to increased apoptosis. These results suggest that mitophagy acts as a mechanism of initial adaptation of cell survival. However, persistent mitochondrial damage induces extensive and lethal mitophagy, autophagic stress, and autophagic permeabilization leading to cell death by apoptosis [61].

5.2. Pregabalin

The postsynaptic NMDA receptors can alter the presynaptic transport of the vesicles that contain neurotransmitters through the NO pathway that diffuses to the presynaptic membrane and alters traffic of the vesicles [67].

5.3. Co-enzyme Q10 (CoQ10)

The CoQ10, a small lipophilic molecule located in the internal mitochondrial membrane, transfers reducing equivalents of the complexes I and II to the complex III of the mitochondrial respiratory chain. The CoQ10 is crucial for the efficiency of the mitochondrial chain, and there is existing evidence that reports CoQ10 as affecting the expression of genes involved in the inflammatory pathways [62]. The presence of mitochondrial dysfunction has been proposed as a relevant fact in the pathogenesis of FM [63]. The mitochondria generate energy primarily in the form of an electrochemical proton gradient that fuels the production of ATP, ion transport, and metabolism. The mitochondria are the primary sources of ROS in the complexes I and III, together with CoQ10 [64]. Management with CoQ10 could be useful as an alternative treatment in FM; however, more studies are needed to confirm whether the beneficial effect is real. More detailed studies through analysis in double blind placebo-controlled clinical trials are required on the effect of CoQ10 in bodily fluids and/or muscle biopsies [65]. In a study by Alcocer-Gomez E et al. included four patients with FM who measured the visual analogue scale (pain, fatigue and sleep), the Generalized Pain Index, the symptom severity scale and the Scl-90-R using the FM Impact Questionnaire High-performance liquid chromatography the CoQ10 content of patients with FM, and the authors found that CoQ10 in the four patients had defiecincy before the treatment, and after the treatment with CoQ10 patients showed significant improvement in clinical symptoms [66].

6. Antioxidants

Antioxidants, like the superoxide dismutase (SOD), catalase, and the glutathione peroxidase (GPx), are enzymes of the defense system that work to prevent oxidative stress through inactivation of the ROS. The SOD enzyme eliminates the damaging effects of the free radicals through the conversion of the radical O^{2-} into hydrogen peroxide (H_2O_2), and the GPx converts H_2O_2 into oxygen and water [67]. The principle intracellular antioxidant enzymes, copper, zinc-SOD (Cu-Zn-SOD) in the cytoplasm, and the manganese-SOD (MnSOD) in the mitochondria, specifically reduce the O^{2-} radicals to H_2O_2. Normally, there is an equilibrium between the ROS and the antioxidants in the cell, in the membranes, and in the extracellular space. However, the antioxidants are overwhelmed by the excessive production of ROS. The ROS attack the polyunsaturated fatty acids of the membrane producing LPO, resulting in alteration to the membrane permeability and changes to the membrane potential. The measurement of thiobarbituric acid reactive substances (TBARS), MDA, or 4-hydroxynonenal is the most common method applied to measure LPO [68]. The central nervous system is especially sensitive to ROS due to its high content of lipids compared to other areas of the body (**Figure 1**) [34].

6.1. Melatonin

Pain is a dynamic phenomenon resultant of the activity of the endogenous system of excitation and inhibition of pain. The efficiency of the system in FM has been related to the quality of sleep [69]. The relationship between pain and quality of sleep is supported on a neurobiological basis by the neurotransmitters involved: norepinephrine, serotonin, and dopamine [70]. The effect of melatonin on pain has been demonstrated in studies on inflammatory pain in experimental animals with neuropathic pain [71, 72] and in acute and chronic pain in clinical studies [73, 74]. Since the most frequent complaints in patients with FM are sleep alterations, fatigue, and chronic pain, these symptoms could be a consequence of the disruption of melatonin secretion [75]. Additionally, there is information that the serum levels of the precursors to melatonin (tryptophan and serotonin) are diminished in patients with FM [76]. The deficiency of melatonin in FM could explain the lack of reparative sleep and could be a mechanism involved in the regulation of dysfunctional pain [77]. There have been reports of studies which suggest that melatonin increases the effect of the descending pain inhibitory system, which involves anatomical connections between cortical regions and the brainstem in the human brain [78]. Therefore, the restoration of melatonin could be an additional mechanism to explain the discrepancy of its effect compared to amitriptyline. In a phase II randomized controlled clinical trial, it was demonstrated that the exogenous administration of 10 mg every 24 h of melatonin augmented the endogenous inhibitory system of pain regulation, evaluated by a numerical scale (0–10), and demonstrated that the association between melatonin with amitriptyline gave better results than the amitriptyline alone, as determined by the visual analog pain scale [79]. Another randomized trial demonstrated that the administration of melatonin alone or in combination with fluoxetine (3–5 mg/day) was efficient in treating FM [80]. However, clear and conclusive evidence from clinical trials or prospective cohorts with prolonged follow-up on the effect of melatonin in patients suffering from FM is still lacking. Melatonin behaves as a free radical scavenger and therefore as a potent antioxidant. Melatonin has physical–chemical advantages over other antioxidant molecules. It is a hormone that is found naturally in the body. Melatonin molecules enter all subcellular organs and compartments. Melatonin detoxifies up to 10 Free Radicals [81]. Compared with other antioxidants, melatonin has equal or better efficacy in the protection of tissues from oxidative lesions such as vitamin C and E. Another inherent feature of melatonin is mitochondrial membrane selectivity and may be the most interesting advantage of pineal hormone [82]. Even melatonin is an effective antioxidant in the prevention of hepatotoxicity induced by amitriptyline [83].

7. Vitamins

Vegetarian diets seem to alleviate some symptoms of FM due to a low content of fat and proteins, high levels of fiber, vitamin C, beta-carotenes, minerals (magnesium, potassium, zinc, and selenium), and antioxidants [49].

In the first controlled pilot study to establish the safety and feasibility of intravenous treatment of micronutrients based on water-soluble vitamins and minerals in FM (Myer's cocktail), the authors reported that the majority of subjects experienced alleviation compared to baseline symptomatology, but they did not observe significant differences between the therapy and the placebo, considering the relationship uncertain between the placebo and micronutrients in FM [84]. According to the Brazilian Society of Rheumatology, the ingestion of sugar, salt, fat, and alcohol should be reduced, and the ingestion of fiber, fruits, vegetables, and fluids increased, in order to avoid the appearance of chronic degenerative illnesses and obesity [85]. Specific micronutrients like calcium (Ca) and magnesium (Mg) are important for proper muscular contraction, and the increase in tryptophan intake can be beneficial in the synthesis of serotonin [86]. The combination of vitamins and minerals can reduce the doses of analgesics and improve the sensation of pain in patients with FM [87]. In the majority of subjects with FM, an inadequate intake of vitamin C is observed. In 2003, Richard et al. demonstrated that the prolonged use of analgesics can augment the excretion of potassium and vitamin C causing anemia from iron deficiency [88]. In the study by Sakarya et al., the authors evaluated blood levels of antioxidant vitamins and Mg in FM patients, and they correlated them with clinical parameters without finding a correlation between the levels of vitamins A, C, E, and Mg with pain severity, functional capacity, and depression. The authors suggest that based on the results, the poor intake of these nutrients does not necessarily signify low blood levels [89]. Folate and vitamin B12 are essential for the regulation of the central nervous system, and their deficiency can result in peripheral neuropathic pain. Vitamin C deficiency can cause myalgia and bone pain, and a deficiency of vitamin D can cause muscle-skeletal pain [90]. The fatigue present in FM seems to have similarities to the manifestations of mild thiamine deficiency [91]. Various similarities have been reported between FM and thiamine deficiency, which include irritability, frequent headache, fatigue, muscular weakness, irritable bowel syndrome, and sleep disturbances. Studies have been published where anomalies in thiamine metabolism have been demonstrated in FM, and investigating thiamine deficiency together with the consumption of alcohol has been suggested in FM patients [92]. The administration of large quantities of oral thiamine increases the blood concentration to levels where the passive transport restores the normal glucose metabolism, and then the normal glucose metabolism of all the organs returns to normal values and symptoms are reduced. It is recommended to prescribe the permanent use of high doses of thiamine in FM [93]. Vitamins A, E, and C are potent nonenzymatic antioxidants [94]. Vitamins A and E are essential fat-soluble vitamins, are the primary chain antioxidants in body tissues, are considered the first line of defense against LPO, they protect the cell membranes early on when the activity of free radicals increases [95]. Vitamin C is the main water-soluble vitamin and is a free radical purifier that transforms vitamin E to its active form [96]. Magnesium (Mg) is a mineral that plays an important role in ATP synthesis and functions in adequate muscle metabolism [97]. Serum levels of Mg have been investigated in FM to reveal etiopathology [98]. Vitamin C is capable of accelerating the degradation of intra- and extracellular proteins targeting lysosomal lumen by autophagic and heterophagic pathways. Vitamin C decreased and stabilized the intra-lysosomal acid pH at values that resulted in maximal activation of the lysosomal hydrolases [99].

7.1. Vitamin D

Vitamin D is a hormone essential for maintaining homeostasis of the muscle-skeletal system. Vitamin D deficiency has been proposed as a factor associated with generalized chronic pain. The majority of vitamin D is produced naturally in the skin after exposure to ultraviolet B light (UVB) producing 25-hydroxyvitamin D (25-OHD). Vitamin D undergoes hydroxylation of the active form 1,25-dihydroxyvitamin D (1,25-OHD) in the liver and kidneys. Age, latitude, time of day, season, skin pigmentation, adiposity, smoking, and amount of exposure to sunlight directly affect the production of vitamin D in the skin [100]. People who are at risk of vitamin D deficiency include people with dark skin, obesity, the elderly, those with chronic degenerative illnesses, or those with disabilities who have little exposure to sunlight [101]. The active form of vitamin D, 1,25-OHD, acts in the cell nucleus (genomic effects caused by gene over-regulation) and the cell membranes (nongenomic effects that cause rapid response) in more than 30 tissues and organs [102]. The muscles are a target organ for the metabolites of vitamin D because they contain receptors for vitamin D identified in the muscle tissues in humans and animals on producing genomic effects that alter calcium, phosphate, and the metabolism of phospholipids [103]. These changes are important for the normal, functional development of the skeletal musculature. There is evidence that the ingestion of vitamin D improves muscle strength and functional capacity. It should be considered that vitamin D decreases in elderly populations, and supplementation is necessary [104]. Recent studies have centered on the potential therapeutic implications of vitamin D and its deficiency, in the regulation of chronic pain processing in FM, through the interactions of central and peripheral complexes. The primary functional scenario of the interaction is based on the presence of the vitamin D receptor and the 1α-hydroxylase (enzyme that converts the 25-hydroxyvitamin D by hydroxylation to the active 1,25 di-hydroxyl-vitamin D (1,25 (OH) 2D3) in many areas of the human central nervous system, among which are: the prefrontal cortex, the amygdala, the raphe, the gelatinous substance, the cerebellum, the hippocampus, the cingulate cortex, the substance *nigra,* the thalamus, and the hypothalamus [105]. Both the receptor and the enzyme have been found in neuronal and glial cells [106]. The general characteristics of hypovitaminosis D are body pain, especially in the shoulder, the thoracic cavity, and lumbar and pelvic regions. The biological relationship between generalized chronic pain and vitamin D deficiency continues to be an interesting investigative topic. Patients with FM could have vitamin D deficiencies due to the characteristics of their pain, poor mobility, or the associated depression that decreases free time exposed to sunlight, or by the increase in adiposity that favors the decrease in vitamin D synthesis. Therefore, the participation of the 1,25-OHD in the regulation of the immune system could be involved in vitamin D deficiency and muscular pain [107]. A systematic review that sought evidence of an association between FM and vitamin D deficiency was inconclusive, without finding improvement in muscular pain after supplementation. However, patients with concurrent risk factors between FM and other pathologies like osteoporosis should be tested in case a vitamin D deficiency is found that would favor muscle strength [108]. The search between vitamin D deficiency and the presence of FM remains an inconclusive matter.

8. Conclusion

In conclusion, oxidative stress, mitochondrial dysfunction, autophagy, multivitamin deficiencies, and the imbalance between oxidants and antioxidants are an intriguing and clinically attractive topic to elucidate the state and progression of FM. Pharmacological treatment alone is insufficient for the majority of patients who suffer from FM syndrome. It is recommended to approach treatment in a multidisciplinary way in clinical practice. Moderate physical activity and the supplementation/ingestion of antioxidants could be beneficial in regulating the oxidative state.

Conflicts of interest

There are no conflicts of interest to report.

This study did not receive any funding.

http://dx.doi.org/10.5772/intechopen.70695

Author details

Alejandra Guillermina Miranda-Díaz* and Simón Quetzalcóatl Rodríguez-Lara

*Address all correspondence to: kindalex1@outlook.com

Department of Physiology, Institute of Clinical and Experimental Therapeutics, University Health Sciences Centre, University of Guadalajara, Guadalajara, Jalisco, México

References

[1] Gerdle B, Björk J, Cöster L, Henriksson K, Henriksson C, Bengtsson A. Prevalence of widespread pain and associations with work status: A population study. BMC Musculoskeletal Disorders. 2008;**9**:102

[2] Bennett RM, Jones J, Turk DC, Russell IJ, Matallana L. An internet survey of 2,596 people with fibromyalgia. BMC Musculoskeletal Disorders. 2007;**8**:27

[3] Heymann RE, Paiva Edos S, Helfenstein M Jr, Pollak DF, Martinez JE, Provenza JR, Paula AP, Althoff AC, Souza EJ, Neubarth F, Lage LV, Rezende MC, de Assis MR, Lopes ML, Jennings F, Araújo RL, Cristo VV, Costa ED, Kaziyama HH, Yeng LT, Iamamura M, Saron TR, Nascimento OJ, Kimura LK, Leite VM, Oliveira J, de Araújo GT, Fonseca MC. Brazilian consensus on the treatment of fibromyalgia. Revista Brasileira de Reumatologia. 2010;**50**:56-66

[4] Tornero MJ, Sanmartí SR, Rodríguez VV, Martín ME, Marenco-de la Fuente JL, González AI, Muñoz FS, Gómez-Reino CJ, Carreño PL, Batlle GE, Balsa CA, Andreu JL, Alvaro-Gracia JM, LJA M, Loza SE. Update of the consensus statement of the Spanish Society of Rheumatology on the management of biologic therapies in rheumatoid arthritis. Reumatologia Clinica. 2010;**6**(1):23-36

[5] Wolfe F, Ross K, Anderson J, Russell IJ, Hebert L. The prevalence and characteristics of fibromyalgia in the general population. Arthritis and Rheumatism. 1995;**38**:19-28

[6] Wolfe F, Smythe HA, Yunus MB, Bennett RM, Bombardier C, Goldenberg DL, Tugwell P, Campbell SM, Abeles M, Clark P, Fam AG, Farber SJ, Fiechtner JJ, Franklin CM, Gatter RA, Hamaty D, Lessard J, Lichtbroun AS, Masi AT, Mccain GA, Reynolds WJ, Romano TJ, Russell IJ, Sheon RP. The American College of Rheumatology 1990 criteria for the classification of fibromyalgia. Report of the multicenter criteria committee. Arthritis and Rheumatism. 1990;**33**:160-172

[7] Bellato E, Marini E, Castoldi F, Barbasetti N, Mattei L, Bonasia DE, Blonna D. Fibromyalgia syndrome: Etiology, pathogenesis, diagnosis, and treatment. Pain Research and Treatment. 2012;**2012**:426130

[8] Gavi MB, Vassalo DV, Amaral FT, Macedo DC, Gava PL, Dantas EM, Valim V. Strengthening exercises improve symptoms and quality of life but do not change autonomic modulation in fibromyalgia: A randomized clinical trial. PloS One. 2014;**9**(3):e90767

[9] Ozgocmen S, Ozyurt H, Sogut S, Akyol O. Current concepts in the pathophysiology of fibromyalgia: The potential role of oxidative stress and nitric oxide. Rheumatology International. 2006;**26**(7):5855-5897

[10] Buskila D, Sarzi-Puttini P. Biology and therapy of fibromyalgia: Genetics aspects of fibromyalgia síndrome. Arthritis Research & Therapy. 2006;**8**:218-222

[11] Bradley LA. Pathophysiology of fibromyalgia. The American Journal of Medicine. 2009;**122**:1-13

[12] Yunus MB, Khan MA, Rawlings KK, Green JR, Olson JM, Shah S. Genetic linkage analysis of multicase families with fibromyalgia syndrome. The Journal of Rheumatology. 1999;**26**:408-412

[13] Staud R. Fibromyalgia pain: Do we know the source? Current Opinion in Rheumatology. 2004;**16**(2):157-163

[14] Melzack R. Evolution of the neuromatrix theory of pain. The Prithvi Raj Lecture: Presented at the Third World Congress of World Institute of Pain, Barcelona 2004. Pain Practice. 2005;**5**(2):85-94

[15] Wolfe F. Fibromyalgia: The clinical syndrome. Rheumatic Diseases Clinics of North America. 1989;**15**:1-18

[16] Kulshreshtha P, Gupta R, Yadav RK, Bijlani RL, Deepak KK. Effect of low-dose amitriptyline on autonomic functions and peripheral blood flow in fibromyalgia: A pilot study. Pain Medicine. 2012;**13**(1):131-136

[17] Davies KJ. Oxidative stress: The paradox of aerobic life. Biochemical Society Symposium. 1995;**61**:1-31

[18] Sánchez A, Calpena AC, Clares B. Evaluating the oxidative stress in inflammation: Role of melatonin. International Journal of Molecular Sciences. 2015;**16**(8):16981-17004

[19] Rodríguez-Lara SQ, Cardona-Muñoz EG, Ramírez-Lizardo EJ, Totsuka-Sutto SE, Castillo-Romero A, García-Cobián TA, García-Benavides L. Alternative interventions to prevent oxidative damage following ischemia/reperfusion. Oxidative Medicine and Cellular Longevity. 2016;**2016**:1-16. DOI: 10.1155/2016/7190943

[20] Evans PH. Free radicals in brain metabolism and pathology. British Medical Bulletin. 1993;**49**:577-587

[21] Buskila D, Cohen H, Neumann L, Ebstein RP. An association between fibromialgia and the dopamine D4 receptor exón III drepet polymorphism and relationship to novelty seeking peronality traits. Molecular Psychiatry. 2004;**9**:730-731

[22] Esterbauer H, Schaur RJ, Zollner H. Chemistry and biochemistry of 4-hydroxynonenal, malonaldehyde and related aldehydes. Free Radical Biology & Medicine. 1991;**11**:81-128

[23] Clot P, Tabone M, Arico S, Albano E. Monitoring oxidative damage in patients with liver cirrhosis and different daily alcohol intake. Gut. 1994;**35**:1637-1643

[24] Cordero MD, Alcocer-Gómez E, Cano-García FJ, De Miguel M, Carrión AM, Navas P, Sánchez Alcázar JA. Clinical symptoms in fibromyalgia are better associated to lipid peroxidation ñevels in blood mononuclear cells rather than in plasma. PloS One. 2011;**6**(10):e26915

[25] Ghafourifar P, Cadenas E. Mitochondrial nitric oxide synthase. Trends in Pharmacological Sciences. 2005;**26**(4):190-195

[26] Kingwell BA. Nitric oxide-mediated metabolic regulation during exercise: Effect of training in health and cardiovascular disease. The FASEB Journal. 2000;**14**(12):1685-1696

[27] Schulman H. Nitric oxide: A spatial second messenger. Molecular Psychiatry. 1999; **2**:296-299

[28] Ghasemi A, Zahediasl S. Is nitric oxide a hormone? Iranian Biomedical Journal. 2011; **15**(3):59-65

[29] Millan MJ. The induction of pain: An integrative review. Progress in Neurobiology. 1999; **57**:1-164

[30] Lindman R, Hagberg M, Bengtsson A, Henricksson KG, Thornell LE. Capillary structure and mitochondrial volume density in the trapezius muscle of chronic trapezius myalgia, fibromyalgia, and healthy subjects. J Musculoskelet Pain. 1995;**3**:5-22

[31] Lund N, Bengtsson A, Thorborg P. Muscle tissue oxygen pressure in primary fibromialgia. Scandinavian Journal of Rheumatology. 1986;**15**:165-173

[32] Jeschonneck M, Graohmann G, Hein G, Sprott H. Abnormal microcirculation and temperature in skin above tender points in patients with fibromyalgia. Rheumatology. 2000;**39**:917-921

[33] Gronemann ST, Ribel-Madsen S, Bartels EM, Danneskiold-Samsoe B, Bliddal H. Collagen and muscle pathology in fibromyalgia patients. Rheumatology. 2004;**43**:27-31

[34] Chinnery PF, Johnson MA, Wardell TM, Singh-Kler R, Hayes C, Brown DT, Taylor RW, Bindoff LA, Turnbull DM. The epidemiology of pathogenic mitochondrial DNA mutations. Annals of Neurology. 2000;**48**:188-193

[35] DiMauro S, Schon EA. Mitochondrial respiratory-chain diseases. The New England Journal of Medicine. 2003;**348**:2656-2668

[36] Cordero MD, De Miguel M, Moreno Fernández AM, Carmona López IM, Garrido Maraver J, Cotán D, Gómez Izquierdo L, Bonal P, Campa F, Bullon P, Navas P, Sánchez Alcázar JA. Mitochondrial dysfunction and mitophagy activation in blood mononuclear cells of fibromialgia patients: Implications in the pathogenesis of the disease. Arthritis Research & Therapy. 2011;**12**:R17

[37] Cordero MD, Moreno-Fernández AM, deMiguel M, Bonal P, Campa F, Jiménez-Jiménez LM, Ruiz-Losada A, Sánchez-Domínguez B, Sánchez Alcázar JA, Salviati L, and Navas P. Coenzyme Q10 distribution in blood is altered in patients with fibromyalgia. Clinical Biochemistry. 2009;**42**:732-735

[38] Kalyan-Raman UP, Kalyan-Raman K, Yunus MB, Masi AT. Muscle pathology in primary fibromyalgia syndrome: A light microscopic, histochemical and ultrastructural study. The Journal of Rheumatology. 1984;**11**:808-813

[39] Sánchez-Domínguez B, Bullón P, Román-Malo L, Marín-Aguilar F, Alcocer-Gómez E, Carrión AM, Sánchez-Alcazar JA, Cordero MD. Oxidative stress, mitochondrial dysfunction and, inflammation common events in skin of patients with fibromyalgia. Mitochondrion. 2015;**21**:69-75

[40] Glick D, Barth S, Macleod KF. Autophagy: Cellular and molecular mechanisms. The Journal of Pathology. 2010;**2010**(221):3-12

[41] Cuervo AM. Autophagy: In sickness and in health. Trends in Cell Biology. 2004;**14**:70-77

[42] Scherz-Shouval R, Shvets E, Fass E, Shorer H, Gil L, Elazar Z. Reactive oxygen species are essential for autophagy and specifically regulate the activity of Atg4. The EMBO Journal. 2007;**26**:1749-1760

[43] Jin S. Autophagy, mitochondrial quality control and oncogenesis. Autophagy. 2006;**2**: 80-84

[44] Nakatogawa H, Suzuki K, Kamada Y, Ohsumi Y. Dynamics and diversity in autophagy mechanisms: Lessons from yeast. Nature Reviews. Molecular Cell Biology. 2009; **10**:458-467

[45] Saftig P, Beertsen W, Eskelinen EL. LAMP-2 a control step for phagosome and autophagosome maturation. Autophagy. 2008;**4**:510-512

[46] Axe EL, Walker SA, Manifava M, Chandra P, Roderick HL, Habermann A, Griffiths G, Ktistakis NT. Autophagosome formation from membrane compartments enriched in phosphatidylinositol 3-phosphate and dynamically connected to the endoplasmic reticulum. The Journal of Cell Biology. 2008;**182**:685-687

[47] Mizushima N. Autophagy: Process and function. Genes & Development. 2007;**21**: 2861-2287

[48] Gomes LC, Scorrano L. Mitochondrial morphology in mitophagy and macroautophagy. Biochimica et Biophysica Acta. 1833;**2013**:205-212

[49] Kim I, Rodriguez-Enriquez S, Lemasters JJ. Selective degradation of mitochondria by mitophagy. Archives of Biochemistry and Biophysics. 2007;**462**:245-253

[50] Oezel L, Then H, Jung AL, Jabari S, Bonaterra GA, Wissniowski TT, Önel SF, Ocker M, Thieme K, Kinscherf R, Di Fazio P. Fibromyalgia syndrome: Metabolic and autophagic processes in intermittent cold stress mice. Pharmacology Research & Perspectives. 2016;**4**(5):e00248

[51] Rodriguez-Hernandez A, Cordero MD, Salviati L, Artuch R, Pineda M, Briones P, Gomez Izquierdo L, Cotan D, Navas P, Sanchez-Alcazar JA. Coenzyme Q deficiency triggers mitochondria degradation by mitophagy. Autophagy. 2009;**5**:19-32

[52] Cordero MD De Miguel M, Fernández AMM, López IMC, Maraver JG, Cotán D, Izquierdo LG, Bonal P, Campa F, Bullon P, Navas P, Alcázar JAS Mitochondrial dysfunction and mitophagy activation in blood mononuclear cells of fibromyalgia patients: Implications in the pathogenesis of the disease. Arthritis Research & Therapy. 2010;**12**(1):R17

[53] Hassett AL, Gevirtz RN. Nonpharmacologic treatment for fibromyalgia: Patient education, cognitive-behavioral therapy, relaxation techniques, and complementary and alternative medicine. Rheumatic Diseases Clinics of North America. 2009;**35**:393-407

[54] Donaldson MS, Speight N, Loomis S. Fibromyalgia syndrome improved using a mostly raw vegetarian diet: An observational study. BMC Complementary and Alternative Medicine. 2001;**1**:7

[55] Turk DC, Okifuji A, Sinclair JD, Starz TW. Differential responses by psychosocial subgroups of fibromyalgia syndrome patients to an interdisciplinary treatment. Arthritis Care and Research. 1998;**11**(5):397-404

[56] Kia S, Choy E. Update on Treatment Guideline in fibromyalgia syndrome with focus on pharmacology. Biomedicines. 2017;**5**(2): pii:E20

[57] Eich W, Häuser W, Friedel E, Klement A, Herrmann M, Petzke F, Offenbächer M, Schiltenwolf M, Sommer C, Tölle T, Henningsen P. Fibromyalgia syndrome. Definition, classification, clinical diagnosis and prognosis. Zeitschrift für Rheumatologie. 2008;**67**(8):665-666 668-672, 674-676

[58] Carette S, Bell MJ, Reynolds WJ, Haraoui B, McCain GA, Bykerk VP, Edworthy SM, Baron M, Koehler BE, Fam AG, et al. Comparison of amitriptyline, cyclobenzaprine, and placebo in the treatment of fibromyalgia. A randomized, double-blind clinical trial. Arthritis and Rheumatism. 1994;**37**:32-40

[59] Scudds RA, McCain GA, Rollman GB, Harth M. Improvements in pain responsiveness in patients with fibrositis after successful treatment with amitriptyline. The Journal of Rheumatology. Supplement. 1989;**19**:98-103

[60] Nishishinya B, Urrútia G, Walitt B, Rodriguez A, Bonfill X, Alegre C, Darko G. Amitriptyline in the treatment of fibromyalgia: A systematic review of its efficacy. Rheumatology. 2008;**47**:1741-1174

[61] Villanueva-Paz M, Cordero MD, Pavón AD, Vega BC, Cotán D, De la Mata M, Oropesa-Ávila M, Alcocer-Gomez E, de Lavera I, Garrido-Maraver J, Carrascosa J, Zaderenko AP, Muntané J, de Miguel M, Sánchez-Alcázar JA. Amitriptyline induces mitophagy that precedes apoptosis in human HepG2 cells. Genes & Cancer 2016;**7**(7-8):260-277

[62] Schmelzer C, Lindner I, Rimbach G, Niklowitz P, Menke T, Döring F. Functions of coenzyme Q10 in inflammation and gene expression. BioFactors. 2008;**32**:179-183

[63] Cordero MD, de Miguel M, Moreno-Fernández AM. Mitochondrial dysfunction in fibromialgia and its implication in the pathogenesis of disease. Medicina Clínica (Barcelona) 2011;**136**(6):252-256

[64] Turunen M, Olsson J, Dallner G. Metabolism and function of coenzyme Q. Biochimica et Biophysica Acta. 1660;**2004**:171-199

[65] Quinzii CM, Lopez LC, Von-Moltke J, Naini A, Krishna S, Schuelke M, Salviati L, Navas P, Dimauro S, Hirano M. Respiratory chain dysfunction and oxidative stress correlate with severity of primary CoQ10 deficiency. The FASEB Journal. 2008;**22**:1874-1885

[66] Alcocer-Gómez E, Cano-García FJ, Cordero MD. Effect of coenzyme Q10 evaluated by 1990 and 2010 ACR diagnostic criteria for fibromyalgia and SCL-90-R: Four case reports and liberature review. Nutrition. 2013;**29**(11-12):1422-1425

[67] Battin EE, Brumaghim JL. Antioxidant activity of Sulfur and selenium: A review of reactive oxygen species scavenging, glutathione eeroxidase, and metal-binding antioxidant mechanisms. Cell Biochemistry and Biophysics. 2009;**55**:1-23

[68] Söğüt S, Zoroğlu SS, Ozyurt H, Yilmaz HR, Ozuğurlu F, Sivasli E, Yetkin O, Yanik M, Tutkun H, Savaş HA, Tarakçioğlu M, Akyol O. Changes in nitric oxide levels and antioxidant enzyme activities may have a role in the pathophysiological mechanisms involved in autism. Clinica Chimica Acta. 2003;**331**:111-117

[69] Paul-Savoie E, Marchand S, Morin M, Bourgault P, Brissette N, Rattanavong V, Cloutier C, Bissonnette A, Potvin S. Is the deficit in pain inhibition in fibromyalgia influenced by sleep impairments? Open Rheumatology Journal. 2012;**6**:296-302

[70] Wood PB, Glabus MF, Simpson R, Patterson JC. Changes in gray matter density in fibromyalgia: Correlation with dopamine metabolism. The Journal of Pain. 2009;**10**:609-618

[71] Laste G, Vidor L, de Macedo IC, Rozisky JR, Medeiros L, de Souza A, Meurer L, de Souza IC, Torres IL, Caumo W. Melatonin treatment entrains the rest-activity circadian rhythm in rats with chronic inflammation. Chronobiology International. 2013;**30**:1077-1088

[72] Esposito E, Cuzzocrea S. Antiinflammatory activity of melatonin in central nervous system. Current Neuropharmacology. 2010;**8**:228-242

[73] Caumo W, Torres F, Moreira NL, Auzani JA, Monteiro CA, Londero G, Ribeiro DF, Hidalgo MP. The clinical impact of preoperative melatonin on postoperative outcomes in patients undergoing abdominal hysterectomy. Anesthesia and Analgesia. 2007;**105**:1263-1271

[74] Schwertner A, Conceição Dos Santos CC, Costa GD, Deitos A, de Souza A, de Souza IC, Torres IL, da Cunha Filho JS, Caumo W. Efficacy of melatonin in the treatment of endometriosis: A phase II, randomized, double-blind, placebo-controlled trial. Pain. 2013;**154**:874-881

[75] Bazzichi L, Rossi A, Giacomelli C, Bombardieri S. Exploring the abyss of fibromyalgia biomarkers. Clinical and Experimental Rheumatology. 2010;**28**:S125-S130

[76] Yunus MB. Fibromyalgia and overlapping disorders: The unifying concept of central sensitivity syndromes. Seminars in Arthritis and Rheumatism. 2007;**36**:339-356

[77] Wikner J, Hirsch U, Wetterberg L, Röjdmark S. Fibromyalgia–a syndrome associated with decreased nocturnal melatonin secretion. Clinical Endocrinology. 1998;**49**:179-183

[78] Hadjipavlou G, Dunckley P, Behrens TE, Tracey I. Determining anatomical connectivities between cortical and brainstem pain processing regions in humans: A diffusion tensor imaging study in healthy controls. Pain. 2006;**123**:169-178

[79] de Zanette SA, Vercelino R, Laste G, Rozisky JR, Schwertner A, Machado CB, Xavier F, de Souza IC, Deitos A, Torres IL, Caumo W. Melatonin analgesia is associated with improvement of the descending endogenous pain-modulating system in fibromyalgia: A phase II, randomized, double-dummy, controlled trial. BMC Pharmacology and Toxicology. 2014;**15**:1-14

[80] Hussain SA, Al-Khalifa II, Jasim NA, Gorial FI. Adjuvant use of melatonin for treatment of fibromyalgia. Journal of Pineal Research. 2011;**50**:267-271

[81] Tan DX, Manchester LC, Terron MP, Flores LJ, Reiter RJ. One molecule, many derivatives: A never-ending interaction of melatonin with reactive oxygen and nitrogen species. Journal of Pineal Research. 2007;**42**:28-42

[82] Dragicevic N, Copes N, O'Neal-Moffitt G, Jin J, Buzzeo R, Mamcarz M, Tan J, Cao C, Olcese JM, Arendash GW, et al. Melatonin treatment restores mitochondrial function in Alzheimer's mice: A mitochondrial protective role of melatonin membrane receptor signaling. Journal of Pineal Research. 2011;**51**:75-86

[83] Taziki S, Sattari MR, Dastmalchi S, Eghbal MA. Cytoprotective effects of melatonin against amitriptyline-induced toxicity in isolated rat hepatocytes. Advanced Pharmaceutical Bulletin. 2015;**5**(3):329-334

[84] Ali A, Njike VY, Northrup V, Sabina AB, Williams AL, Liberti LS, Perlman AI, Adelson H, Katz DL. Intravenous micronutrient therapy (Myers' cocktail) for fibromyalgia: A placebo-controlled pilot study. Journal of Alternative and Complementary Medicine. 2009;**15**(3):247-257

[85] Sociedade Brasileira de Reumatologia – SBR. Dieta. Available from: http://www.fibromialgia.com.br/novosite/index.php?modulo=pacientes_artigos&id_mat_mat=11&id_mat=10. [Accessed: June 16, 2017]

[86] Kim YS, Kim KM, Lee DJ, Kim BT, Park SB, Cho DY, Suh CH, Kim HA, Park RW, Joo NS. Women with fibromyalgia have lower levels of calcium, magnesium, iron and manganese in hair mineral analysis. Journal of Korean Medical Science. 2011;**26**(10):1253-1257

[87] Batista ED, Andretta A, de Miranda RC, Nehring J, Dos Santos Paiva E, Schieferdecker ME. Food intake assessment and quality of life in women with fibromyalgia. Revista Brasileira de Reumatologia (English Edition). 2016;**56**(2):105-110

[88] Rokyta R, Holecek V, Pekárkova I, Krejcová J, Racek J, Trefil L, Yamamotová A. Free radicals after painful stimulation are influenced by antioxidants and analgesics. Neuro Endocrinology Letters. 2003;**24**(5):304-309

[89] Sakarya ST, Akyol Y, Bedir A, Canturk F. The relationship between serum antioxidant vitamins, magnesium levels, and clinical parameters in patients with primary fibromyalgia síndrome. Clinical Rheumatology. 2011;**30**(8):1039-1043

[90] Bell RF, Borzan J, Kalso E, Simonnet G. Food, pain, and drugs: Does it matter what pain patients eat? Pain. 2012;**153**(10):1993-1996

[91] World Health Organization. Thiamine deficiency and its prevention and control in major emergencies. Geneva: Department of Nutrition for Heath and Development, WHO; 1999 Report No: WHO/NHD/99.13

[92] Monroe BA. Fibromyalgia—A hidden link? Journal of the American College of Nutrition. 2013;**1998**:300-303

[93] Lonsdale D. A review of the biochemistry, metabolism and clinical benefits of thiamin (e) and its derivatives. Evidence-Based Complementary and Alternative Medicine. 2013;**2006**:49-59

[94] Nazıroğlu M, Şimşek M, Kutlu M. Moderate exercise with dietary vitamin C and E combination protects streptozotocin-induced oxidative damage to the blood and improves fetal outcomes in pregnant rats. Clinical Chemistry and Laboratory Medicine. 2004;**42**:511-517

[95] Packer L, Landvik S. Vitamin E in biological systems. Advances in Experimental Medicine and Biology. 1990;**264**:93-103

[96] Sies H, Stahl W. Vitamins E and C, β-carotene, and other carotenoids as antioxidants. The American Journal of Clinical Nutrition. 1995 Dec;**62**(6):1315S-1321S

[97] Romano TJ, Stiller JW. Magnesium deficiency in fibromyalgia syndrome. Journal of Nutritional Medicine. 1994;**4**:165-166

[98] Sendur OF, Tastaban E, Turan Y, Ulman C. The relationship between serum trace element levels and clinical parameters in patients with fibromyalgia. Rheumatology International. 2008;**28**:1117-1121

[99] Martin A, Joseph JA, Cuervo AM. Stimulatory effect of vitamin C on autophagy in glial cells. Journal of Neurochemistry. 2002;**82**(3):538-549

[100] Laaksi I, Ruohola JP, Tuohimaa P, Auvinen A, Haataja R, Pihlajamäki H, Ylikomi T. An association of serum vitamin D concentrations <40 nmol/L with acute respiratory tract infection in young Finnish men. The American Journal of Clinical Nutrition. 2007;**86**:714-717

[101] McCabe PS, Pye SR, Mc Beth J, Lee DM, Tajar A, Bartfai G, Boonen S, Bouillon R, Casanueva F, Finn JD, Forti G, Giwercman A, Huhtaniemi IT, Kula K, Pendleton N, Punab M, Vanderschueren D, Wu FC, O'Neill TW, EMAS Study Group. Low vitamin D and the risk of developing chronic widespread pain: Results from the European male ageing study. BMC Musculoskeletal Disorders. 2016;**17**:32

[102] Norman AW. From vitamin D to hormone D: Fundamentals of the vitamin D endocrine system essential for good health. The American Journal of Clinical Nutrition. 2008;**88**:491S-4499

[103] Ceglia L. Vitamin D and its role in skeletal muscle. Calcified Tissue International. 2013;**92**(2):151-156

[104] Pfeifer M, Begerow B, Minne HW, Suppan K, Fahrleitner-Pammer A, Dobnig H. Effects of a long-term vitamin D and calcium supplementation on falls and parameters of muscle function in community-dwelling older individuals. Osteoporosis International. 2009;**20**:315-322

[105] Jirikowski GF, Kaunzner UW, Dief Ael E, Caldwell JD. Distribution of vitamin D binding protein expressing neurons in the rat hypothalamus. Histochemistry and Cell Biology. 2009;**131**:365-370

[106] Shipton EA, Shipton EE. Vitamin D and pain: Vitamin D and its role in the aetiology and maintenance of chronic pain states and associated comorbidities. Pain Research and Treatment. 2015;**2015**:904967

[107] Atherton K, Berry DJ, Parsons T, Macfarlane GJ, Power C, Hyppönen E. Vitamin D and chronic widespread pain in a white middle-aged British population: Evidence from a cross-sectional population survey. Annals of the Rheumatic Diseases. 2009;**68**:817-822

[108] Daniel D, Pirotta MV. Fibromyalgia. Should we be testing and treating for vitamin D deficiency? Australian Family Physician. 2011;**40**(9):712-716

Nonpharmacologic Treatment for Fibromyalgia

Fatmanur Aybala Koçak and Emine Eda Kurt

Additional information is available at the end of the chapter

http://dx.doi.org/10.5772/intechopen.70515

Abstract

Fibromyalgia is a common musculoskeletal pain condition associated with chronic widespread pain, tenderness at various points on the body, fatigue, and sleep abnormalities. Individuals with fibromyalgia often have comorbid anxiety, depression, and/or other pain syndromes. Research into pharmacologic remedies for fibromyalgia has demonstrated efficacy for a variety of agents, but pharmacology is only one piece of the puzzle when it comes to successful management of fibromyalgia. Nonpharmacological treatments, complementary and alternative medicines, and therapies can support alleviating fibromyalgia symptoms.There are many studies with regard to these treatment options.

Keywords: fibromyalgia, nonpharmacologic treatment

1. Introduction

Fibromyalgia (FM) has been defined as a chronic and common pain disorder and is associated with comorbid symptoms such as fatigue, nonrestorative sleep, poor balance, cognition and memory problems, psychological distress, and physical function impairment [1]. The life quality is also reduced in FM [2]. It is affecting approximately 2% of the general population [3]. FM is also an expensive and controversial condition. It has been associated with significantly higher costs for the individual and society [4]. However, current data do not enable identification of distinct factors in the etiology and pathophysiology of fibromyalgia syndrome [5]. Also, an important problem in FM patients is the low compliance rate which, in the case of most patients, depends on an inadequate clinical response and on the difficulty in making a correct clinical characterization of patients [6]. Among the treatment options for FM management, there are pharmacological as well as nonpharmacologic therapies (supplementary and alternative medical treatments included) [7]. Numerous studies were reported about different nonpharmacologic treatment options [8–10].

In this chapter, nonpharmacological treatment options will be explained in light of the last published guidelines.

2. Education and goal setting

The diagnosis of FM has positive influences on the management of this disease and leads to decrease in primary care visit, diagnostic tests and prescriptions. The nest stage is the training of patients. When the patient is convinced that the disease is not life-threatening, the anxiety will decrease [11]. The training and detailed goal setting are extremely important. Training on the treatment must be provided to the patient and his/her family as well. Acknowledging of the pain and the effects of this pain in his/her life is important. The patient must also be told to be active in his/her rehabilitation period, and it must be emphasized that she/he is not alone in this process. In this step, concrete goals must be set during the treatment period [12]. Mentioning the positive expectations from the treatment period and the prognosis and the participation of the patient are, again, extremely important. It is also useful to tell patients that there will be good days and bad days and that the treatment will decrease the effects of the symptoms but not completely eliminate the disease. It is extremely important that the patients are careful about the sleep hygiene, exercise schedule and some other nonpharmacologic modalities [11].

Strong evidence shows that patient training is effective in the FM management. In a randomized-controlled study, untreated controls were compared with trained FM patients and positive outcomes were reported [13]. The training was generally provided in groups like lectures with printed materials, discussions with groups and demonstrations. The duration of the trainings lasted between 6 and 17 sessions. The positive outcomes of the trainings included improvement in pain, sleep quality, fatigue, self-efficacy, and quality of life. Positive outcomes lasted between 3 and 12 months. In a study in which 100 patients were included, a multidisciplinary training program was applied for 1–1/2 days, and important positive improvements were reported it terms of Fibromyalgia Impact Questionnaire (FIQ) total score, pain scores, fatigue, morning tiredness, stiffness, anxiety, and depression in the 1-month follow-up [13, 14].

According to some clinicians, labeling FM in itself would deteriorate the symptoms, but a prospective study showed that the labeling, i.e., the diagnosis, did not have any adverse effects, on the contrary, it improved function over 18 months [15].

There are several studies in which well-controlled trials were reported as well as some other studies that reported that they could not find statistically significant superiority over other intervention methods when compared with the trained control group [16]. Burckhardt et al. [17] provided training to FM patients in one group, physical training condition and training to another group, and included delayed treatment waitlist controls in another third group [17]. They reported improved measurements in terms of physical activity in the active treatment groups [18].

If the patients are prone to be trained on self-management of the FM, a training and multiprofessional or multimodal program is the most important first-step action to involve the patients in the planned therapeutic activities. If such a program is not possible, an informed physician can provide patient education, and for detailed nonpharmacologic treatments, a specialist may also be consulted [18, 19].

3. Exercises

McLoughlin et al. [20] reported that many female patients with FM are active at a less level when compared with healthy women whose ages match [20]. They have low perceived functional ability. They also demonstrate impaired physical performance [21]. There are many reports that described positive effects of various types or combined exercises on patients with FM [22]. Pain in FM patients may be associated with the central nervous system (CNS) pain-processing abnormalities including central sensitization and insufficient pain inhibition, peripheral tissues, as well as muscles, which might contribute to chronic pain via initiating and/or maintaining central sensitization [23]. In this way, exercise is expected to contribute to pain via muscle microtrauma process, repair and adaptation, which are associated with normal-acute exercise and exercise training. It has been reported in previous studies that there are metabolic outcomes in muscle tissues, which is consistent with deconditioning [24]. Some of these findings might be normalized by aerobic and strength training-induced metabolic adaptations, which contribute to improvements in pain [25]. In addressing conditions experienced by FM patients, exercise training was reported to be used successfully [8].

Although there are studies mentioning the efficiency of short-term aerobic exercises, the level of evidence for these studies is low. Effects on pain and tender points were determined to be at an insignificant level in statistical terms. In terms of the secondary outcomes such as depression, fatigue and sleep, the evidence is not clear on the effects of aerobic exercise on depression (in this respect, two studies reported medium/large effects [26]). There is no evidence that aerobic exercise prescribed at American College of Sports Medicine levels had effects on fatigue in FM patients [27]. Despite the fact that a meta-analysis shows that aerobic exercise has a positive effect on well-being and physical function, several factors moderated our appraisal. It has been demonstrated that aerobic and strength training improves depression in individuals that have depression at clinical level [28]. Moderate exercise can be beneficial for sleep in people with sleep complaints. It is also visible in training-related improvements in cardiorespiratory fitness. This situation suggests that fatigue may also be improved because as the maximal aerobic capacity of a person improves, that person will perform daily life activities at lower absolute percentages of maximal capacity [22]. Kurt et al. conducted a randomized study and reported that the FIQ score, sleep quality, total myalgic score, and depression scores of the group that received only aerobic exercise treatment improved after 15 sessions; however, in the third month follow-up, it was observed that the measurements regressed to the values that were present before the treatment. In recent studies, it has been reported that especially combined exercises or the combinations of exercise and other treatment options are more efficient [29].

According to a Cochrane compilation conducted on the efficiency of resistance exercises in FM patients, it has been reported that moderate- and moderate- to high-intensity resistance training improves pain, tenderness, muscle strength, and multidimensional function in FM patients, and it is obvious that the level of evidence for these studies is low. In addition, it has also been reported that resistance exercises are superior to flexibility exercises in terms of wellness, FM symptoms, and physical fitness; however, aerobic exercises are more successful than resistance exercises [8]. In an 8-week exercise program in which aerobic exercises and muscle strengthening exercises were compared, it was reported that fitness, depression, pain, sleep, fatigue, tender point count, and quality of life were improved in FM patients in both exercise groups, and no differences at statistically significant level were observed between the two exercise types [30].

There are exercise recommendations given in the past years such as American Pain Society (APS: 2005), (2) Association of the Scientific Medical Societies in Germany (AWMF: 2012), (3) Canadian Pain Society (CPS: 2013; also used in the United Kingdom), and (4) European League Against Rheumatism (EULAR: 2016) guidelines related to FM. APS, CPS, and AWMF assigned the highest ranking of recommendation for aerobic exercises [31]. In EULAR 2016 FM management guide, the proof levels of aerobic and stretching exercises are given as A in Ia Proof Level. However, according to the previous studies, it has also been reported that none of the two exercises was superior to the other one [10].

Besides these, especially in the last decade, extensive research was conducted on low-impact aerobics, flexibility, stretching, strength training exercise technique spectra, and some traditional exercise techniques such as Tai Chi, chi gong, yoga, and Nordic walk. In a more recent cohort study, it has been reported that Tai-Chi exercises could be an efficient rehabilitation method for FM in case it was done with the supervision of an expert [32]. It has been reported that Ai-Chi exercises, which are a form of Tai-Chi movements in water, led to reduced pain and improved life quality as well as physical-mental health in FM patients in a 10-week aquatic therapy program [33].

In two randomized-controlled studies, it was reported that Tai Chi had a potential as a useful method in the multidimensional treatment of FM [34]. Furthermore, studies showed improvement at a statistically significant level in static and dynamic balance, and timed get-up-and-go. According to these results, it was shown that functional mobility decreased the falling risk with Tai Chi in functional measurements and minimized difficulties in performing essential daily physical activities [35]. The German Pain Society 2017 guideline in "Complementary and alternative procedures for fibromyalgia syndrome" strongly recommends Qigong, Tai Chi, and yoga for the FM treatment [36].

Fischer-White et al. [37] conducted a compilation study and reported that there was a need for comprehensive yoga instructions, and they stated that the use of yoga in FM was investigated by a limited number of researchers, although there were no adequate proofs [37]. The yoga programs included traditional yoga postures, breathing exercises and meditation. In a study in which 22 FM women patients were included in an 8-week yoga program, improvements were observed in fibromyalgia symptoms and functional deficit [38]. In a controlled study conducted by Ide et al. [39] pranayama (a breathing technique in yoga) was utilized in combination with a range of motion and relaxation exercises in aquatic medium for female FM patients (sessions lasted for 1 h, four times a week, and 4 weeks). Important improvements were shown on several SF-36 and FIQ components together with global pain and dyspnea scores [39].

In recent years, Pilates has become a popular exercise form for healthy people and for people who need rehabilitation. Pilates exercises focus on core strengthening, posture, and coordination of breathing with movement and combines Asian and Western techniques. In 2009, Altan et al. [40] conducted a study and examined the effects of Pilates in 49 female FM patients. They showed improvements in pain scores and FIQ results compared to the control group (home relaxation and stretching exercises); but after an extra 12-week follow-up, no differences were detected between the groups [40]. In a recent randomized controlled study, the Visual Analogue Scale, algometry, Anxiety Inventory, FIQ, and Quality of life score were showed to improve in patients with FM [41].

In a study in which moderate-to-high intensity aerobic exercise by means of Nordic walking and low-intensity walking exercises applied twice a week (in 15 weeks) was compared, the former was found to be a feasible mode of exercise and resulted in improved functional capacity and a decreased level of activity limitations [42]. Mannerkorpi et al. [43] conducted a randomized-controlled study and reported similar results [43]. In a meta-analysis in which the effect of Qigong, which is a Chinese medical exercise combining static/dynamic physical exercises, breathing exercises, and meditation on FM was investigated, it was reported that there were little number of patients and studies on the topic, and although there was a low-quality evidence, Qigong might be a useful approach for FM patients in terms of pain, life quality, and sleep improvements [44].

In a Cochrane compilation in which the aquatic exercise studies were compiled, it was reported in studies that compared study groups and control groups that improvements could be achieved in aquatic exercise group in terms of pain, involvement, and physical functions. When aquatic exercises were compared with land exercises, it was reported that there were no differences at a statistically significant level between the groups, and when aquatic exercises were compared with the Ai-Chi exercises, it was reported that Ai Chi was superior to aquatic exercises for stiffness [45]. Recently, a randomized-controlled study, which includes both aquatic therapy and land-based therapy (warm-up, proprioceptive exercises, stretching, and relaxation periods), was reported. In a program of the study being applied for 3 days a week for 3 months, improvements were determined in both groups in terms of pain and balance, but no significant differences were detected between the groups [46]. Andrade et al. [47] reported that aquatic physical training with standardized intensities did not cause significant changes in body composition but was effective in promoting increased VO_2 at peak cardiopulmonary exercise test in women with FM [47]. The purposes of physical activity and exercise training include improving physical fitness and function together with the symptoms of fibromyalgia, and optimizing health, because a sedentary lifestyle and deconditioning are associated with the symptoms of fibromyalgia [20]. Moreover, a lower percentage of maximum capacity may be achieved in daily activities with more efficiency and the symptoms are less likely to increase [48]. Furthermore, targets depend on baseline body functions and the severity of the symptoms together with individual preferences and motivations [49]. In contrast, in a study, it was reported that nearly 2% of the competitive sport players had FM, which shows that people with FM may be extremely active. Although regular exercises (i.e., aerobic, strength, flexibility) are among the most important elements in the FM management, it is also important that the intensity, duration, incidence, and type of any adverse effects and frequency must be prescribed [50]. Prescribing exercises for FM patients requires extreme care. After a detailed assessment that includes cardiovascular system, a personal exercise program for the target is designed [48]. Although the most prominent exercises are aerobics and stretching exercises in many studies, there is no such thing as "the most proper treatment." Different exercises may be combined in the same séance or in different séances. However, the evidence level on flexibility exercises is low, and they are generally combined with stretching exercises [51].

It has been reported by many authors that the frequency of exercises must be increased gradually starting from low intensity (by using the "*start-low & go-slow*" technique) to achieve at least moderate intensity [52]. Strengthening exercises must be started at lower resistance level of the normal values according to the age. If pain, fatigue and other FM symptoms increase, the duration of exercise session must be decreased. Also, the intensity of the exercises should be increased by 10% within 2 weeks of exercise (without exacerbating the symptoms) [48]. In recent studies, a formula that was computed with heartbeat according to the age in FM patients was developed. In terms of the target heartbeat zones for aerobic training within the anaerobic threshold, a training intensity range was shown to improve cardiorespiratory fitness. In previous studies, authors reported that maximum heartbeat could be predicted by using either $(208 - (0.7 \times \text{age}))$ or $(220 - \text{age})$. They also suggested sedentary individuals with FM to train within the anaerobic threshold at 52–60% of the heartbeat reserve or at 75–85% of the predicted maximum heartbeat [53].

4. Physical treatment modalities

The definition of physical therapies involves all treatments in which a physical activity or technique is used to have therapeutic effects. Such techniques are mostly used in the context of rehabilitation and are used on the basis of their ascertained mechanisms of action (i.e., the activation of the spinal gate, release of endogenous opiates, local metabolic action, etc.) Physical therapies have several types such as thermal (hot and cold), mechanical, light, electrical, and magnetic stimulation. Each of these has its own mechanism of action; however, peer-reviewed evidence of their effectiveness in FM is missing. Recent reviews have reported nonhomogeneous results, while some reviews are cautious in stating efficacy based only on few randomized-controlled trials. It is strongly suggested to conduct more studies to show a long-term, effective intervention for managing the FM symptoms [54]. Other reviews that have anecdotal evidence or small-scale observational physiotherapy studies report that physical therapies can be effective for various symptoms [55, 56].

4.1. Heat and cold

Although local cold therapy application with ice cubes or cooling sprays is useful in other muscle pains, they do not have any influence in FM. Cold sprays are applied with stretch-spray techniques. On the other hand, whole body cryotherapy at −67°C seems to have some short-term effect on some active trigger points and on the intensity of the pain. There are no data available about the long-term efficacy [56, 57].

Superficial heat and deep infrared heat, ultrasound application and the local thermal effect induced by stroking massages were reported to be useful for FM patients [58, 59]. The real efficacy of both superficial and deep heat is still a topic for further studies [56].

4.2. Balneotherapy, mud-pack/bath, hydrotherapy

The exact mechanisms of immersion of the body in mineral/thermal water or applying mud, which alleviates FM symptoms, are not understood adequately. It is considered that this effect stems from a combination of mechanical, thermal and chemical factors [60].

To discriminate between nonspecific mechanisms of simple bathe in hot water (hydrotherapeutic, in a broader sense), specific mechanisms (hydromineral and crenotherapeutic) depending on chemical and physical properties of the water are used. Buoyancy, resistance, immersion, and temperature together play important roles in this mechanism. Hot stimuli increase the threshold of pain and produce analgesia on nerve endings. A relief in muscle spasms is achieved via gamma fibers in muscle spindles and the descending pain inhibitory system is activated. The "Gate Theory" claims that relief in pain may stem from the temperature and hydrostatic pressure of water on the skin [61]. The absorption of minerals dissolved in thermal waters may be influential in the mechanism of balneotherapy [61, 62].

Some previous studies reported that sulfur baths had anti-inflammatory effects. Spa water that includes sulfur is thought to inhibit the production of cytokines especially IL-2 and interferon gamma. It has been claimed by some authors that memory T-cells are the principal targets of waters that are rich in sulfur because they are mainly produced by CD4 lymphocytes. Sulfur-containing water reduces the capacity of memory T-cells to proliferate and therefore the cytokine production, which alters immune response [63].

The exact mechanism of balneotherapy on fibromyalgia is not clear yet. Ardiç et al. [64] showed decreased levels of anti-inflammatory markers interleukin 1 (IL-1), prostaglandin E2, and leukotriene B4 after 15 sessions of balneotherapy in 44 FM patients [64]. Furthermore, heat and mineral contents of water have useful effects on body (especially in musculoskeletal, endocrinologic system, and in pain pathways). They also contain increased plasma endorphin and cortisol levels, and are responsible for the activation of diencephalic-pituitary-adrenal axis and decreased plasma levels of several inflammatory mediators (IL-1, IL-6, prostaglandin E2, leukotriene B4, tumor necrosis factor alpha) [29, 61]. Balneotherapy is recommended strongly by AWMF, APS and EULAR for the FM treatment [31]. In EULAR recommendations, it has been stated that without balneotherapy and exercise, hydrotherapy would not have any superiority and both were recommended with weak recommendation level [10]. In a recent comprehensive meta-analysis that investigated the efficiency of balneotherapy in FM patients, it was reported that there was weak evidence on the efficiency of balneotherapy; however, it could be applied as a supplementary treatment together with the basic treatment. It has been observed that the frequency and duration of treatment were taken in different terms in many different studies. There is no standardization on this [65].

In a 2-week study in which Bağdatlı et al. [66] compared the efficiency of balneotherapy and mud-pack, it was reported that Balneotherapy was a more efficient treatment in terms of nonrefreshed awaking, pain intensity, FIQ score, fatigue, stiffness, anxiety, and depression subscales of FIQ in the follow-up measurements 1 month after the treatment [66]. The efficiency of balneotherapy and mud-bath was compared in another randomized-controlled study, and it was reported that both the treatments were influential on FM symptoms; however, the effect of mud-bath lasted more [67]. In a study conducted by Neumann et al., it was reported that balneotherapy had useful effects on FM symptoms and on the life quality of the patients [68].

After the treatment, Evcik et al. [69] reported important improvements in three parameters. It was reported in their study that there were low FIQ scores and some painful points at the sixth month follow-up assessments when they compared the baseline. However, Beck depression scores were increased to near-baseline level [69]. Dönmez et al. [70] also conducted a study and reported that balneotherapy was influential on FIQ scores, sleep disturbance, and on some painful points when compared to the baseline values in the sixth month [70]. In a randomized-controlled study in which combined treatment approaches were compared, it was reported that when balneotherapy and aerobic exercises were applied together with the existing treatment, the FIQ, depression scale, sleep quality, and total myalgic scores were better when compared to the exercise + balneotherapy group, and in addition, the effect duration could last as long as 3 months in terms of sleep quality in a combined therapy [29].

4.3. Electrical stimulation: TENS

Electrical current is the most frequently used physical therapy technique in pain management. Transcutaneous electrical nerve stimulation (TENS) is an electrical current for pain relief applied by means of superficial electrodes applied on skin. Investigators have found positive results with fibromyalgia using TENS [71]. In one review article, it was reported that TENS was a useful methodology to control specific symptoms like localized musculoskeletal pain [55]. On the other hand, it is possible to claim that TENS and related techniques can be useful in treating specific, contingent and localized pains, but they do not have obvious effects on generalized pain syndromes like FM [56].

4.4. Transcranial direct current stimulation (tDCS) and transcranial magnetic stimulation (TMS)

The possibility of central mechanisms in the pathogenesis of FM has led to the idea that transcranial stimulation treatments can be performed. Thus, studies were conducted in FM patients. The tDCS procedure applies a weak current to the scalp, while TMS therapy uses electrical current to produce a magnetic field. Then this magnetic field penetrates to skull to generate an electrical field in the brain of the patient. Stimulation of the primary motor cortex produces antinociceptive effects, while stimulation of the dorsolateral prefrontal cortex has antidepressant effects.

In a review that examined the effectiveness of tDCS and TMS, decrease in pain scores was reported after these treatments, but different results were reported in the number of tender points, in functional assessments, and in depression scales [72]. In a guideline about therapeutic use of tDCS, level B evidence (probable efficacy) was found for FM [73]. In a more recent meta-analysis about the effectiveness of tDCS in FM, it is more likely to control pain and improve general FM-related function in FM patients than sham tDCS [74].

4.5. Laser

The data on using laser in FM are few and conflicting; however, there are some rare studies reporting efficacy. In some studies, it has been reported that there were no effects [75, 76] while in some others, it has been reported that there is a statistically significant reduction in both spontaneous and mechanical pain [77]. It is difficult to compare various treatment protocols because of the varying lengths of emission wave and power across different and nonstandardized protocols [56].

4.6. Biofeedback

There are numerous studies in the literature on biofeedback approaches. Buckelew et al. [78] conducted a study and compared electromyogram (EMG) biofeedback, exercise training, combination treatment (biofeedback and exercise) and an educational/attention control group [78]. Compared to the control group, they reported that patients in the treatment groups showed improvements in some functional and clinical scores. Another controlled trial was conducted in which patients were assigned to either a fitness program or surface EMG, and the authors could not show significant improvement compared to the control group [79]. Although there are contrary results, the findings that are mostly positive suggest that EMG biofeedback may be a preferred treatment option for some patients with FM [18].

In the revised recommendations of EULAR for managing FM, there were two reviews that were conducted about biofeedback. Glombiewski et al. [80] reviewed 7 studies with 321 participants. Treatment sessions varied from 6 to 22. The control therapy consisted of sham biofeedback, attention control, medication and treatment as usual. Biofeedback was influential in reducing the intensity of the pain, although all trials showed poor quality. EULAR has weak opposition about biofeedback [10].

5. Cognitive behavioral therapies

Cognitive behavioral therapies (CBTs) are a combination of cognitive + behavioristic therapies. In cognitive part, such a therapy will ensure that there will occur changes in emotions and behaviors [18]. In this way, several drawbacks like overgeneralizing, magnifying negative aspects, minimizing positive ones and catastrophizing will be eliminated. Such drawbacks will be replaced with realistic and effective considerations, which will eventually decrease emotional stress and self-defeating behavior. Specifically, in FM, the consideration or the expectation of the worst possible outcome has been associated with the severity of the pain, decreased functioning and affective distress in FM [81, 82]. In cognitive therapy step, worries like "*This is the worst pain, and I cannot do anything*" are replaced with statements such as "*Although my pain is worse, there are still things I can do to lessen it.*" Behavioral therapy, on the other hand, unlike the cognitive one, is based on the claim that thoughts and feelings are not as important as operant behaviors, and tries to increase adaptive behavior via positive-negative reinforcement. Behavioral therapy also extinguishes maladaptive behaviors by punishing the patient in such cases. There are several behavioral techniques that might be applied in FM like behavioral activation (getting patients move again), graded exercises (initiating exercise and then activities increasing slowly), activity pacing (not overdoing it on the days when the patient feels well and remaining active on days when the patient feels bad), pain-reducing behaviors (not reinforcing behaviors related with secondary gain), sleep hygiene (identifying the behaviors that are known to disrupt sleep), and learning relaxation techniques for the purpose of lowering stress (for example imagery, breathing, muscle relaxation, etc.) [18].

In general, applying CBT for FM has three steps [83]. Step 1 consists of training in which the participation of the patient in pain management is focused on and the nature of the pain is dealt with. In step 2, there is skill training on pain reduction to improve functional status and sleep quality, etc. In Step 3, these skills are applied in real-life situations. CBT also involves homework assignments to learn and practice these skills. The "Booster Sessions" also aim the same thing and help to sustain the effects for longer durations [84].

In the revised recommendations of EULAR for managing FM there were 5 reviews that included 30 trials and at least 2031 participants about CBT. Although the quality of individual trials was reported as being weak in general, in one quality review, there were 23 trials comprising >2000 patients [85]. Cognitive behavioral therapies (CBTs) were effective in reducing pain and disability after the treatment when compared with the controls. The results lasted for longer durations. EULAR proposes behavioral therapies as weak [10].

6. Traditional and complementary medicine

The requirement of traditional and complementary medicine (TCM) processes is very common in patients with chronic diseases for which conventional therapies have failed to obtain a cure all around the world. The rheumatologic disorders are one of the most common causes of admission to the TCM practitioners. The TCM usage rate of patients with FM reaches almost 100% [86, 87].

6.1. Acupuncture

Acupuncture is a traditional Chinese medicine form. Needles are placed at various predefined points on the body. It has many effects including reducing pain. It is claimed to work by reducing the inflammation, causing endorphin release, and creating a calmer mind [88]. Many studies showed its use in reducing pain in FM and other pain types when compared to no treatment or sham acupuncture [89]. It has been shown that acupuncture decreases the number and intensity of painful spots. It also modifies neurohormonal parameters [56].

In a clinical study, 70 patients underwent electroacupuncture. It was reported that there was 70% improvement in some parameters in the intervention group against 4% in the sham acupuncture group [90].

In the revised recommendations of EULAR for managing FM, there were eight reviews about acupuncture. In one high-quality review, it was reported that acupuncture, when used together with the standard therapy, resulted in a 30% improvement in pain scores. Electric acupuncture was also associated with improvements in pain and fatigue. Some mild and transient adverse events were also reported. The active mechanism of acupuncture has not been clarified, and the evidence supporting the use of real vs. sham acupuncture is less consistent. EULAR proposes acupuncture as weak [10].

6.2. Manual therapy/massage/chiropractic

Manual treatments are hands-on therapies used to increase motion range and to decrease pain and swelling. Tissue and muscles relaxation along with stretching exercises is the commonly used manual treatments. Proprioceptive neuromuscular facilitation is used to increase range of motion and strength. Pain leads to immobilization, which further leads to soft tissue (fascia, tendons, ligaments etc.) restriction that can create abnormal strain pattern that can crowd or pull the osseous structures out of proper alignment resulting in compression of joints, which produces pain and/or dysfunction. Neural and vascular structures can also be compressed causing neurological or ischemic conditions. Shortening of the myofacial fasicle can limit its functional length, reducing its strength contractile potential or deceleration capacity facilitating positive changes in this system by therapeutic intervention like myofascial release. Mobilizing the restricted fissure can reverse the effects of immobilization provided that it does not last for an excessive period. Movement encourages the collagen fibers to align themselves along the lines of structural stress and improves the balance of glycosaminoglycans and lubricates and hydrates the corrective tissues [91].

Massage is commonly used in TCM therapy in FM patients. Based on the patient survey data, the intervention has been reported with the highest satisfaction levels [18].

A systematic review and meta-analysis examined fatigue, anxiety, depression, and sleep disturbance. They also included studies investigating traditional Chinese massage that was not extensively reviewed previously. Their main result was that massage therapy that lasted more than 5 weeks gave significant improvement in pain, anxiety, and depression [89, 92].

In the revised recommendations of EULAR for managing FM, there were 6 reviews reported including 1 meta-analysis in which there are 9 trials and 404 patients. Methodological problems were noted with all of the studies, only four were at low risk of bias in terms of random allocation. EULAR has a weak opposition about massage [10].

Chiropractic treatments, like massage therapy, have also become a popular modality in FM patients. Few randomized-controlled trials were reported in FM patients using chiropractic modalities [18, 56]. In the revised recommendations of EULAR for managing FM, there were three reviews about chiropractics. The most recent compilation summarized three studies [93]. The studies were of poor quality and lacked robust data. EULAR has strong opposition about chiropractic treatments [10].

6.3. Meditative movement/mindfulness/mind-body therapy

"Mind and body therapy" is a heterogeneous term that means as "meditative movement therapy" or "complementary and alternative exercise." The goal is to improve the flow of qi (the life energy) through the body with purposeful hand and body movements. A review of studies demonstrated improvements after 6 months compared to baseline in patients with FM. However, the studies had significant methodological issues and variability [94]. Tai Chi is another mind-body technique with specific movements. A meta-analysis that included seven studies evaluated Tai Chi for FM that showed improvements in some symptoms [89, 95].

In the revised recommendations of EULAR for managing FM, there were six reviews focusing on qigong, yoga, Tai Chi, or a combination of them. However, there was inadequate evidence for individual recommendations. EULAR proposes meditative movement as weak [10].

There were 6 reviews that included 13 trials and 1209 participants about mindfulness/mind-body therapy in the EULAR revised recommendations. One recent review provided evidence that mindfulness-based stress reduction resulted in improvements in pain compared with usual care. However, these effects were considered to be biased. EULAR proposes mindfulness/mind-body therapy as weak [10].

6.4. Guided imagery/hypnotherapy

Although hypnosis is one of the oldest therapies for pain, interest in hypnosis for controlling chronic pain rose only in the last decade. Hypnosis is defined as a state of consciousness involving focused attention and reduced peripheral awareness and is characterized by an enhanced capacity for response to suggestion [96]. Imagery is defined as a dynamic, psycho-physiological process in which a person imagines and experiences an internal reality in the absence of external stimuli. These images can be initiated by the patient or guided by a therapist. In a systematic review conducted on evaluating the efficacy, acceptability and safety of guided imagery/hypnosis (GI/H) in FM, randomized-controlled trials comparing GI/H with controls were analyzed. The main outcomes were ≥50% pain relief, ≥20% improvement of health-related quality of life, psychological distress, disability, acceptability and safety at the end of therapy and a 3-month follow-up. There were 7randomized controlled trials (RCTs) with 387 subjects that were included into a comparison of GI/H vs. controls. There was a benefit from GI/H compared to the controls at the end of the therapy [97]. In the revised recommendations of EULAR for managing FM, hypnotherapy evaluation was considered weak [10].

7. Conclusion

FM is a common musculo-skeletal disorder and is otherwise known by unexplained chronic widespread pain, a lower pain threshold, high tender point count (tenderness on examination at specific, predictable anatomic sites known as tender points), sleep disturbances, fatigue, headache, irritable bowel syndrome, morning stiffness, paresthesia of the extremities, frequent psychological distress, and depressed mood [98]. For these reasons, FM has a negative effect on work capacity, family life, social functions, and life quality [7]. Typically, management of fibromyalgia is multidisciplinary. Furthermore, the treatment of the patients must be organized individually after the detailed examination. There are many nonpharmacologic treatment options available in the treatment of fibromyalgia. When this disease is thought to last for a lifetime, increasing the quality of life of patients should be the primary goal. It should

http://dx.doi.org/10.5772/intechopen.70515

concentrate first on nonpharmacologic modalities. This is in view of accessibility, cost, safety and patient preference. It is considered that in addition to the existing standard treatment modality of the patient, the treatment may be more efficient and the burden of medication might be reduced with the selection of the best nonpharmacologic treatment option for the patient.

Among these nonpharmocologic treatment methods, exercise therapy, balneotherapy, cognitive behavioral therapies, acupuncture, and meditative movement/mindfulness/mind-body therapies are more effective treatment methods according to the evidence-based medicine approach. These are summarized in **Table 1**. In case of severe disability, combination therapies should be performed.

Nonpharmacologic therapies	Which symptoms improved after treatment
Exercise therapy	
Aerobic exercise	Pain [10, 29, 30], physical functions [10, 29], global well-being [30], emotional distress/depression [28–30], fatigue [22, 30], number of tender points [29, 30], sleep disturbance [29, 30], decreased quality of life [30]
Strengthening exercise	Pain [8, 10, 30], physical functions [8, 10], global well-being [8, 30], emotional distress/depression [28, 30], fatigue [22, 30], number of tender points [8, 29, 30], sleep disturbance [29, 30], decreased quality of life [30]
Tai Chi exercises/Ai-chi exercises/yoga	Pain [32, 39],decreased quality of life [32, 33, 39], loss of balance [35], physical functions [39]
Balneotherapy	Pain [10, 66–70], fatigue [66–68], stiffness [66], physical functions [66, 67, 69, 70], emotional distress/depression/anxiety [66, 68, 69], decreased quality of life [67, 68], sleep disturbance [67, 68, 70], headache/gastrointestinal disturbances [67, 68], number of tender points [67, 69]
Cognitive behavioral therapies	Pain [10, 18], disability [10, 18], emotional distress/depression/anxiety/ maldaptive thoughts [18], fatigue [18]
Acupuncture	Pain [10, 56, 88, 89], fatigue [10, 88], stiffness [88, 89], global well-being [88], number of tender points [89]
Meditative movement/ mindfulness/mind-body therapies	Sleep disturbance [10, 89, 94, 95], fatigue [10, 94, 95], emotional distress [10, 94], pain [10, 89, 94, 95]

*According to the evidence-based results of guidelines, systematic reviews and meta-analyses.

Table 1. Most effective* nonpharmacological therapies for fibromiyalgia.

Author details

Fatmanur Aybala Koçak and Emine Eda Kurt*

*Address all correspondence to: eedakurt@gmail.com

Medical Faculty, Department of Physical Medicine and Rehabilitation, Ahi Evran University, Kırşehir, Turkey

References

[1] Wolfe F, Clauw DJ, Fitzcharles M-A, et al. The American College of Rheumatology preliminary diagnostic criteria for fibromyalgia and measurement of symptom severity. Arthritis Care and Research. 2010;**62**:600-610

[2] Mease PJ, Arnold LM, Crofford LJ, et al. Identifying the clinical domains of fibromyalgia: Contributions from clinician and patient delphi exercises. Arthritis Care and Research. 2008;**59**:952-960

[3] Häuser W, Ablin J, Perrot S, Fitzcharles MA. Management of fibromyalgia: Practical guides from recent evidence-based guidelines. Polish Archives of Internal Medicine. 2017;**127**(1):47-56

[4] Sicras-Mainar A, Rejas J, Navarro R, et al. Treating patients with fibromyalgia in primary care settings under routine medical practice: A claim database cost and burden of illness study. Arthritis Research and Therapy. 2009;**11**(2):R54

[5] Üçeyler N, Burgmer M, Friedel E, et al. Etiology and pathophysiology of fibromyalgia syndrome: Updated guidelines 2017, overview of systematic review articles and overview of studies on small fiber neuropathy in FMS subgroups. Schmerz 2017;**31**:239-245. DOI: 10.1007/s00482-017-0202-5

[6] Bazzichi L, Giacomelli C, Consensi A, et al. One year in review 2016: Fibromyalgia. Clinical and Experimental Rheumatology. 2016;**34**:145-149

[7] Bennett RM.The rational management of Fibromyalgia patients. Rheumatic Diseases Clinics of North America. 2002;**28**:181-199

[8] Busch AJ, Webber SC, Richards RS, et al. Resistance exercise training for fibromyalgia. Cochrane Database of Systematic Reviews. 2013;**12**:CD010884

[9] Theadom A, Cropley M, Smith HE, Feigin VL, McPherson K. Mind and body therapy for fibromyalgia. Cochrane Database of Systematic Reviews. 2015;**4**:CD001980. DOI: 10.1002/14651858.CD001980

[10] Macfarlane GJ, Kronisch C, Dean LE, et al. EULAR revised recommendations for the management of fibromyalgia. Annals of the Rheumatic Diseases. 2017;**76**:318-328

[11] Hawkins RA. Fibromyalgia: A clinical update. The Journal of the American Osteopathic Association. 2013;**113**:680-689

[12] Turk DC, Vierck CJ, Scarbrough E, Crofford LJ, Rudin NJ. Fibromyalgia: Combining pharmacological and nonpharmacological approaches to treating the person, not just the pain. The Journal of Pain. 2008;**9**:99-104

[13] Goldenberg DL, Burckhardt C, Crofford L. Management of fibromyalgia syndrome. Journal of the American Medical Association. 2004;**292**:2388-2395

[14] Pfeiffer A, Thompson JM, Nelson A, et al. Effects of a 1.5-day multidiscplinary outpatient treatment program for fibromyalgia: A pilot study. American Journal of Physical Medicine and Rehabilition. 2003;**82**:186-191

[15] White K, Nielson WR, Harth M, et al. Does the label "fibromyalgia" alter health status, function and health service utilization?: A prospective within-group comparison in a community cohort of adults with chronic widespread pain. Arthritis and Rheumatism. 2002;**47**:260-265

[16] Goossens ME, Rutten-van Mölken MP, Leidl RM, et al. Cognitive-educational treatment of fibromyalgia: A randomized clinical trial. I. Clinical effects. The Journal of Rheumatology. 1996;**23**:1237-1245

[17] Burckhardt CS, Mannerkorpi K, Hedenberg L, et al. A randomized, controlled clinical trial of education and physical training for women with fibromyalgia. The Journal of Rheumatology. 1994;**21**:714-720

[18] Hassett AL, Gevirtz RN. Nonpharmacologic treatment for fibromyalgia: patient education, cognitive-behavioral therapy, relaxation techniques, and complementary and alternative medicine. Rheumatic Diseases Clinics of North America. 2009;**35**: 393-407

[19] Rooks DS, Gautam S, Romeling M, et al. Group exercise, education, and combination self-management in women with fibromyalgia: A randomized trial. Archives of Internal Medicine. 2007;**167**:2192-2200

[20] McLoughlin MJ, Colbert LH, Stegner AJ, Cook DB. Are women with fibromyalgia less physically active than healthy women? Medicine and Science in Sports and Exercise. 2011;**43**:905-912

[21] Jones CJ, Rutledge DN, Aquino J. Predictors of physical performance and functional ability in people 50+ with and without fibromyalgia. Journal of Aging and Physical Activity. 2010;**18**:353-368

[22] Busch AJ, Barber KA, Overend TJ, Peloso PMJ, Schachter CL. Exercise for treating fibromyalgia syndrome. Cochrane Database of Systematic Reviews. 2007;**4**:CD003786. DOI: 10.1002/14651858.CD003786

[23] Staud R. Biology and therapy of fibromyalgia: Pain in fibromyalgia syndrome. Arthritis Research & Therapy. 2006;**8**(3):208

[24] Elvin A, Siosteen AK, Nilsson A, Kosek E. Decreased muscle blood flow in fibromyalgia patients during standardised muscle exercise: A contrast media enhanced colour Doppler study. European Journal of Pain. 2006;**10**(2):137-144

[25] Deschenes MR, Kraemer WJ. Performance and physiologic adaptations to resistance training. American Journal of Physical Medicine & Rehabilitation. 2002;**81**(11 Suppl): 3-16

[26] Gowans SE, deHueck A, Voss S, Silaj A, Abbey SE. Six month and one-year follow up of 23 weeks of aerobicnexercise for individuals with fibromyalgia. Arthritis Care & Research. 2004;**51**(6):890-898

[27] Schachter CL, Busch AJ, Peloso P, Sheppard MS. The effects of short vs long bouts of aerobic exercise in sedentary women with fibromyalgia: A randomized controlled trial. Physical Therapy. 2003;**83**(4):340-358

[28] Brosse AL, Sheets ES, Lett HS, Blumenthal JA. Exercise and the treatment of clinical depression in adults: Recent findings and future directions. Sports Medicine. 2002;**32** (12):741-760

[29] Kurt EE, Koçak FA, Erdem HR, Tuncay F, Kelez F. Which non-pharmacological treatment is more effective on clinical parameters in patients with fibromyalgia: Balneotherapy or aerobic exercise? Archives of Rheumatology. 2016;**31**(2):162-169. DOI: 10.5606/ArchRheumatol. 2016.5751

[30] Bircan Ç, Karasel SA, Akgün B, El Ö, Alper S. Effects of muscle strengthening versus aerobic exercise program in fibromyalgia. Rheumatology International. 2008;**28**:527-532

[31] Thieme K, Mathys M, Turk DC. Evidenced-based guidelines on the treatment of patients: Are they consistent and ıf not, why not? have effective psychological treatments been overlooked? Journal of Pain. 2016;**27**. DOI: 10.1016/j.jpain.2016.12.006

[32] Maddali Bongi S, Paoletti G, Calà M, Del Rosso A, El Aoufy K, Mikhaylova S. Efficacy of rehabilitation with Tai Ji Quan in an Italian cohort of patients with Fibromyalgia Syndrome. Complementary Therapies in Clinical Practice. 2016;**24**:109-115. DOI: 10.1016/j. ctcp.2016.05.010

[33] Perez-De la Cruz S, Lambeck J. Effects of a programme of aquatic Ai Chi exercise in patients with fibromyalgia. A pilot study. Revista De Neurologia. 2015;**60**(2):59-65

[34] Jones KD, Sherman CA, Mist SD, Carson JW, Bennett RM, Li F. A randomized controlled trial of 8-form Tai chi improves symptoms and functional mobility in fibromyalgia patients. Clinical Rheumatology. 2012;**31**:1205-1214

[35] Wang C, Schmid CH, Rones R, et al. A randomized trial of tai chi for fibromyalgia. The New England Journal of Medicine. 2010;**363**:743-754

[36] Langhorst J, Heldmann P, Henningsen P, et al. Complementary and alternative procedures for fibromyalgia syndrome: Updated guidelines 2017 and overview of systematic review articles. Schmerz. 2017;**31**(3):289-295. DOI: 10.1007/s00482-017-0206-1

[37] Fischer-White TG, Anderson JG, Taylor AG. An ıntegrated methodology to assess compliance with delphi survey key components of yoga ınterventions for musculoskeletal conditions as applied in a systematic review of fibromyalgia studies. Explore (NY). 2016;**12**(2):100-112. DOI: 10.1016/j.explore.2015.12.003

[38] Carson JW, Carson KM, Jones KD, et al. A pilot randomized controlled trial of the Yoga of awareness program in the management of fibromyalgia. Pain. 2010;**151**:530-539

[39] Ide MR, Laurindo LMM, Rodrigues-Junior AL, Tanaka C. Effect of aquatic respiratory exercise-based program in patients with fibromyalgia. International Journal of Rheumatic Diseases. 2008;**11**:131-140

[40] Altan L, Korkmaz N, Bingol U, Gunay B. Effect of pilates training on people with fibromyalgia syndrome: A pilot study. Archives of Physical Medicine and Rehabilitation. 2009;**90**(12):1983-1988. DOI: 10.1016/j.apmr.2009.06.021

[41] Ekici G, Unal E, Akbayrak T, Vardar-Yagli N, Yakut Y, Karabulut E. Effects of active/ passive interventions on pain, anxiety, and quality of life in women with fibromyalgia: Randomized controlled pilot trial. Women & Health. 2017;**57**(1):88-107

[42] Jones KD. Nordic walking in fibromyalgia: A means of promoting fitness that is easy for busy clinicians to recommend. Arthritis Research & Therapy. 2011;**13**(1):103. DOI: 10. 1186/ar3225

[43] Mannerkorpi K, Nordeman L, Cider A, Jonsson G. Does moderate-to-high intensity Nordic walking improve functional capacity and pain in fibromyalgia? A prospective randomized controlled trial. Arthritis Research & Therapy. 2010;**12**(5):189. DOI: 10.1186/ar3159

[44] Lauche R, Cramer H, Häuser W, Dobos G, Langhorst J. A systematic review and meta-analysis of qigong for the fibromyalgia syndrome. Evidence-based Complementary and Alternative Medicine. 2013;**2013**:635182. DOI: 10.1155/2013/635182

[45] Bidonde J, Busch AJ, Webber SC, et al. Aquatic exercise training for fibromyalgia. Cochrane Database of Systematic Reviews. 2014;**10**:CD011336. DOI: 10.1002/14651858.CD011336

[46] Rivas Neira S, Pasqual Marques A, Pegito Pérez I, Fernández Cervantes R, Vivas Costa J. Effectiveness of aquatic therapy vs land-based therapy for balance and pain in women with fibromyalgia: A study protocol for a randomised controlled trial. BMC Musculo-skeletal Disorders. 2017;**18**(1):22. DOI: 10.1186/s12891-016-1364-5

[47] Andrade CP, Zamunér AR, Forti M, França TF, Tamburús NY, Silva E. Oxygen uptake and body composition after aquatic physical training in women with fibromyalgia: A randomized controlled trial. European Journal of Physical and Rehabilitation Medicine. 2017. DOI: 10.23736/S1973-9087.17.04543-9

[48] Jones KD, Liptan GL. Exercise interventions in fibromyalgia: Clinical applications from the evidence. Rheumatic Diseases Clinics of North America. 2009;**35**:373-391

[49] Nijs J, Mannerkorpi K, Descheemaeker F, Van Houdenhove B. Primary care physical therapy in people with fibromyalgia: Opportunities and boundaries within a monodisciplinary setting. Physical Therapy. 2010;**90**:1815-1822

[50] Inanici F, Ozdemir O, Aydog T, et al. The frequency of fibromyalgia in sport professionals. Rheumatology International. 2011;**31**(8):1121-1122. doi: 10.1007/s00296-010-1567-2.

[51] Cazzola M, Atzeni F, Salaffi F, et al. Which kind of exercise is best in fibromyalgia therapeutic programmes? A practical review. Clinical and Experimental Rheumatology. 2010;**28**:117-124

[52] Lemos MC, Valim V, Zandonade E, Natour J. Intensity level for exercise training in fibromyalgia by using mathematical models. BMC Musculoskeletal Disorders. 2010;**11**:54

[53] Busch AJ, Webber SC, Brachaniec M,et al. Exercise therapy for fibromyalgia. Current Pain and Headache Reports 2011;**15**:358-367. DOI: 10.1007/s11916-011-0214-2

[54] Gur A. Physical therapy modalities in management of fibromyalgia. Current Pharmaceutical Design. 2006;**12**:329-359

[55] Offenbächer M, Stucki G. Physical therapy in the treatment of fibromyalgia. Scandinavian Journal of Rheumatology. 2000;**113**:78-85

[56] Casale R, Cazzola M, Arioli G, et al. Non pharmacological treatments in fibromyalgia. Reumatismo. 2008;**60**:59-69

[57] Gutenbrunner C, Englert G, Neuen-Lahusen M, Gehrke A. Controlled study on effects of cold chamber exposures (−67°C, 3 min] in fibromyalgia. Akt Rheumatology. 1999;**24**:77-84

[58] Citak-Karakaya I, Akbayrak T, Demirturk F et al. Short and long-term results of connective tissue manipulation and combined ultrasound therapy in patients with fibromyalgia. Journal of Manipulative and Physiological Therapeutics. 2006;**29**:524-528

[59] Almeida TF, Roizenblatt S, Benedito-Silva AA, Tufik S. The effect of combined therapy (ultrasound and interferential current) on pain and sleep in fibromyalgia. Pain. 2003;**104**: 665-672

[60] Fioravanti A, Cantarini L, Guidelli GM, Galeazzi M. Mechanisms of action of spa therapies in rheumatic diseases: What scientific evidence is there? Rheumatology International. 2011; **31**:1-8

[61] Guidelli GM, Tenti S, De Nobili E, Fioravanti A. Fibromyalgia syndrome and spa therapy: Myth or reality? Clinical Medicine Insights Arthritis and Musculoskelet Disorders. 2012;**5**:19-26. DOI: 10.4137/CMAMD.S8797

[62] Kurt EE, Erdem HR, Tuncay F. Balneotherapy in chronic inflammatory rheumatic disease. Journal of Physical Medicine & Rehabilitation Sciences. 2016;**19**(3):167-173

[63] Ghersetich I, Lotti TM. Immunologic aspects: Immunology of mineral water spas. Clinics in Dermatology. 1996;**14**:563-566

[64] Ardiç F, Ozgen M, Aybek H, Rota S, Cubukçu D, Gökgöz A. Effects of Balneotherapy on serum IL-1, PGE2 and LTB4 levels in fibromyalgia patients. Rheumatology International. 2007;**27**:441-446

[65] Naumann J, Sadaghiani C. Therapeutic benefit of Balneotherapy and hydrotherapy in the management of fibromyalgia syndrome: A qualitative systematic review and meta-analysis of randomized controlled trials. Arthritis Research & Therapy. 2014;**16**(4):141. DOI: 10.1136/annrheumdis-2017-211587

[66] Bağdatlı AO, Donmez A, Eröksüz R, Bahadır G, Turan M, Erdoğan N. Does addition of 'mud-pack and hot pool treatment' to patient education make a difference in fibromyalgia

patients? A randomized controlled single blind study. International Journal of Biometeorology. 2015;**59**(12):1905-1911. DOI: 10.1007/s00484-015-0997-7

[67] Bazzichi L, Da Valle Y, Rossi A,et al. A multidisciplinary approach to study the effects of Balneotherapy and mud-bath therapy treatments on fibromyalgia. Clinical and Experimental Rheumatology. 2013;**31**(6 Suppl 79):111-120

[68] Neumann L, Sukenik S, Bolotin A, et al. The effect of Balneotherapy at the Dead Sea on the quality of life of patients with fibromyalgia syndrome. Clinical Rheumatology. 2001;**20**:15-19

[69] Evcik D, Kizilay B, Gökçen E. The effects of Balneotherapy on fibromyalgia patients. Rheumatology International. 2002;**22**:56-59

[70] Dönmez A, Karagülle MZ, Tercan N, et al. SPA therapy in fibromyalgia: A randomised controlled clinic study. Rheumatology International. 2005;**26**:168-172

[71] Sunshine W, Field TF, Quintino O, et al. Fibromyalgia benefits from massage therapy and transcutaneous electrical stimulation. Journal of Clinical Rheumatology. 1996;**2**:18-22

[72] Marlow NM, Bonilha HS, Short EB. Efficacy of transcranial direct current stimulation and repetitive transcranial magnetic stimulation for treating fibromyalgia syndrome: A systematic review. Pain Practice. 2013;**13**:131-145

[73] Lefaucheur JP, Antal A, Ayache SS, et al. Evidence-based guidelines on the therapeutic use of transcranial direct current stimulation (tDCS). Clinical Neurophysiology. 2017 Jan;**128**:56-92

[74] Zhu CE, Yu B, Zhang W, et al. Effectiveness and safety of transcranial direct current stimulation in fibromyalgia: A systematic review and meta-analysis. Journal of Rehabilitation Medicine. 2017;**49**:2-9

[75] Matsutani LA, Marques AP, Ferreira EA, et al. Effects of muscle stretching exercises with and without laser therapy at tender points for patients with fibromyalgia. Clinical and Experimental Rheumatology. 2007;**25**:410-415

[76] Waylonis GW, Wilke S, O'Toole D, Waylonis DA, Waylonis DB. Chronic myofascial pain: Management by low-output helium-neon laser therapy. Archives of Physical Medicine and Rehabilitation. 1988;**69**:1017-1020

[77] Gur A, Karakoc M, Nas K, et al. Effects of low power laser and low dose amitriptyline therapy on clinical symptoms and quality of life in fibromyalgia: A single-blind, palcebo-controlled trial. Rheumatology International. 2002;**22**:188-193

[78] Buckelew SP, Conway R, Parker J, et al. Biofeedback/relaxation training and exercise interventions for fibromyalgia: A prospective trial. Arthritis Care and Research. 1998;**11**:196-209

[79] van Santen M, Bolwijn P, Verstappen F, et al. A randomized clinical trial comparing fitness and biofeedback training versus basic treatment in patients with fibromyalgia. The Journal of Rheumatology. 2002;**29**:575-581

[80] Glombiewski JA, Bernardy K, Häuser W. Efficacy of EMG- and EEG-biofeedback in fibromyalgia syndrome: A meta-analysis and a systematic review of randomized controlled trials. Evidence-based Complementary and Alternative Medicine. 2013;**2013**: 962741

[81] Gracely RH, Geisser ME, Giesecke T, et al. Pain catastrophizing and neural responses to pain among persons with fibromyalgia. Brain. 2004;**127**:835-843

[82] Edwards RR, Bingham CO, Bathon J, et al. Catastrophizing and pain in arthritis, fibromyalgia and other rheumatic diseases. Arthritis and Rheumatism. 2006;**55**:325-332

[83] Keefe FJ. Cognitive behavioral therapy for managing pain. Clinical Psychologist. 1996;**49**: 4-5

[84] Friedberg F, Williams DA, Collinge W. Lifestyle-oriented non-pharmacological treatments for fibromyalgia: A clinical overview and applications with home-based technologies. Pain Research. 2012;**5**:425-435

[85] Bernardy K, Klose P, Busch AJ, et al. Cognitive behavioural therapies for fibromyalgia. Cochrane Database of Systematic Reviews. 2013;**10**(9):CD009796. doi: 10.1002/14651858. CD009796

[86] Kibar S. Fibromiyalji Sendromu Tedavisinde Tamamlayıcı Tıp Yöntemleri. Turkiye Klinikleri J PM&R-Special Topics. 2015;**8**:50-56

[87] Wahner-Roedler DL, Elkin PL, Vincent A, et al. Use of complementary and alternative medical therapies by patients referred to a fibromyalgia treatment program at a tertiary care center. Mayo Clinic Proceedings. 2005;**80**:55-60

[88] Deare JC, Zheng Z, Xue CCL, et al. Acupuncture for treating fibromyalgia. Cochrane Database of Systematic Reviews. 2013;**31**(5):CD007070. doi: 10.1002/14651858.CD007070

[89] Chinn S, Caldwell W, Gritsenko K. Fibromyalgia pathogenesis and treatment options update. Current Pain and Headache Reports. 2016;**20**:25

[90] Braz AS, de Paula AP, Diniz Mde F, de Almeida RN. Non-pharmacological therapy and complementary and alternative medicine in fibromyalgia. Revista Brasileira de Reumatologia. 2011;**51**:269-282

[91] Kaur J, Kaur N. Fibromyalgia: Non-pharmacological management. Delhi Psychiatry Journal. 2008;**11**:39-42

[92] Li Y-H, Wang F-Y, Feng C-Q, Yang X-F, Sun Y-H. Massage therapy for fibromyalgia: A systematic review and meta-analysis of randomized controlled trials. PLoS One. 2014;**9**: e89304

[93] Ernst E. Chiropractic treatment for fibromyalgia: A systematic review. Clinical Rheumatology. 2009;**28**:1175-1178

[94] Sawynok J, Lynch M. Qigong and fibromyalgia: Randomized controlled trials and beyond. Evidence-based Complementary and Alternative Medicine. 2014;**2014**:379715

[95] Raman G, Mudedla S, Wang C. How effective is Tai Chi mind-body therapy for fibromyalgia: A systematic review and meta-analysis. Journal of Alternative and Complementary Medicine. 2014;**20**:A66-A66

[96] Elkins GR, Barabasz AF, Council JR, Spiegel D. Advancing research and practice: The revised APA Division 30 definition of hypnosis. The International Journal of Clinical and Experimental Hypnosis. 2015;**63**:1-9

[97] Zech N, Hansen E, Bernardy K, Häuser W. Efficacy, acceptability and safety of guided imagery/hypnosis in fibromyalgia—A systematic review and meta-analysis of randomized controlled trials. European Journal of Pain. 2017;**21**:217-227

[98] Mease P. Fibromyalgia syndrome: Review of clinical presentation, pathogenesis, outcome measures and treatment. The Journal of Rheumatology. 2005;**32**:6-21

Chapter 4

Natural Products as Promising Pharmacological Tools for the Management of Fibromyalgia Symptoms – A Review

Renan Guedes Brito, Priscila Laise Santos,
Marlange Almeida Oliveira, Lícia Tairiny Santos Pina,
Angelo Roberto Antoniolli,
Jackson Roberto Guedes da Silva Almeida,
Laurent Picot, Gokhan Zengin,
Jullyana Souza Siqueira Quintans and
Lucindo José Quintans Júnior

Additional information is available at the end of the chapter

http://dx.doi.org/10.5772/intechopen.70016

Abstract

Fibromyalgia (FM) is the second most common rheumatologic disorder, affecting 5% of the world population, and has a serious effect on the quality of life of patients, as well as an economic impact through lost workdays. This pain syndrome is a common cause of chronic widespread pain and is characterized by reduced pressure pain thresholds with hyperalgesia and allodynia, nonrestorative sleep, fatigue, cognitive dysfunction, and mood disturbances. The pharmacological treatment strategies for FM include the use of antidepressants, calcium channel modulators, muscle relaxants, and analgesics but have shown limited efficacy and therapeutic adherence. Thus, researchers have been seeking potential substances (new chemical entities or through drug repositioning) that could be used for FM treatment. In this context, natural products (NPs) have been shown to be promising pharmacological tools due to the variety of their pharmacological activity and the number of molecular sites available as possible active targets. Recent clinical and preclinical studies have been conducted to verify the possible applicability of NPs such as essential oils (EOs), plants extracts, terpenes, sapogenins, and alkaloids in the treatment of FM. The results have shown that natural products have an analgesic effect in different animal models of FM, probably by activation of inhibitory descending pathways, such as the periaqueductal gray and rostroventromedial medulla. Natural products and their secondary metabolites could therefore be a promising source for FM management. However, translational studies that seek to validate the preclinical studies are scarce, incipient, and lacking an approach focused on the traditional pharmaceutical market.

Keywords: natural products, muscle pain, chronic pain, fibromyalgia, pain

1. Introduction

Fibromyalgia (FM) is a painful syndrome caused by changes in the central nervous system. This syndrome is chronic in nature and is present in about 5% of the world population. Generalized musculoskeletal pain and changes in sensitivity, as well as fatigue in the absence of any organic disease, are presented as clinical aspects. Other important symptoms may manifest in patients with FM such as sleep disturbances and cognitive problems, as well as a variety of psychosomatic symptoms. Patients with FM often complain of tingling, numbness, burning, cutaneous hyperalgesia, momentary pain attacks, and depression [1].

Pathophysiological factors are genetic predisposition, autonomic and emotional dysfunctions, physical or environmental stresses, and neurohormonal and inflammatory dysfunctions [2]. Besides that, ischemia and muscular microtraumas, which result in pain during and after exercise, can be considered favorable for the onset of pain in FM. Elvin et al. [3] studied 10 female fibromyalgic patients and 11 female patients in the control group, using Doppler ultrasound in the infraspinatus muscle during low-intensity exercise. Experimental patients presented muscle ischemia when compared to control patients, perhaps because they evoked reflexes in the muscular sympathetic nervous activity, resulting in vasoconstriction. This may be contributed to pain in FM, which could be resulting from possible microtraumas. An abrupt increase in muscle vascularization during and after dynamic exercise was also observed for patients with FM, which did not occur with static exercise when compared to the control patients. Thus, increased muscle sympathetic nerve activity in the FM group may have resulted in imbalance between vasodilation and sympathetic vasoconstriction.

Areas of the descending pathway of pain, such as the periaqueductal gray (PAG) and rostroventromedial area (RVM), which have mainly opioid and serotonergic activation, respectively, may act in endogenous analgesia. These two areas make connections with the dorsal horn of the spinal cord, modulating the transmission of nociceptive messages [3, 4]. Changes in these areas of the central nervous system (CNS) probably occur due to a neurochemical imbalance, with the glutamatergic, 5-HTergic and opioidergic systems being important targets to control this neurotransmitter fluidity. This results in the classification of FM as a central pain syndrome, also known as "dysfunctional pain," where there are changes in sensitivity such as allodynia (pain due to a stimulus that normally does not cause pain) and hyperalgesia (increased pain of a stimulus that usually causes pain), without any tissue or nervous injury [5–7].

Due to the complexity of its pathophysiology, the treatment of FM is very difficult. Only 30% of the medicines used to treat FM have some positive effect. Some drugs have high costs (financial or in terms of side effects), being possible triggers of collateral effects such as nausea, edema, tachycardia, and with poor therapeutic efficacy [1, 2, 8–12]. In order to better understand the physiopathology as well as to investigate new treatment options for FM, animal models have been developed that mimic some symptoms of this syndrome. Scientists have used a combination of repetitive stimuli applied to the muscle, coupled with stress added to the nociceptive stimuli applied in the muscle to trigger lasting hyperalgesia, which mimics FM (**Table 1**) [13–16].

In the search for new sources of more effective drugs with fewer side effects, scientists have been focusing on the study of different pharmacological approaches including natural products (NPs) due to their promising effects on the CNS. NPs are considered the main source of new chemical entities in the search for new medicines and may be fundamental to the discovery of new drugs for diseases or syndromes that still do not respond adequately to the current available treatments. In this context, an important approach to discover new painkillers has been developed with NPs such as medicinal plants or their secondary metabolites that could modulate painful conditions, including FM [17].

Medicinal plants (MPs) are natural products that have been used in the control of several diseases by the world's population for thousands of years. Popular knowledge about the use of these plants has directed scientists to conduct new research seeking drugs that act on specific targets or multiple molecular sites such as the pathophysiology of FM usually presents [18, 19]. Many drugs that are commonly used in clinical treatment are derived directly or indirectly from MPs and include analgesics such as aspirin (anti-inflammatory nonsteroidal derived from salicylic acid, which was initially extracted from *Salix alba*) and morphine (opioid analgesic derived from *Papaver somniferum*) [20]. As evidence of the importance of natural products, between 2005 and 2010, the Food and Drug Administration (FDA) and the European Medicines Agency (EMA) approved 19 medicines derived from NPs, including trabectedin (Yondelis™) and cannabidiol (Sativex®), for cancer and pain treatment, respectively [21, 22]. Moreover, the growing number of patents to protect new formulations containing NPs demonstrates the importance of these compounds [23].

In relation to FM, some classes of bioactive compounds extracted from medicinal plants have presented analgesic activity described in the literature, such as essential oils [24–26], extracts [27, 28], monoterpenes [29–31], sesquiterpenes [32], saponins [33], and alkaloids (**Figure 1** and **Table 2**) [34].

Author	Animal model	Induction	Similarities with the clinical condition	Limitations of the model
Sluka, Kalra, Moore [35]	Acid saline-induced pain	Two injections of acid saline (pH 4; im) separated by 2–5 days	Widespread and generalized hyperalgesia including the bilateral hind limbs, muscles, paws, and viscera, and anxiety	It is not clear if there are comorbidities such as depression, anxiety, fatigue, or sleep disturbances, as in FM. Unlike what is observed in FM, the model is sensitive to opioids intrathecally
Dina, Levine, Green [36]; Dina, Green, Levine [37]	Hyperalgesic priming model	An acute inflammatory insult (carrageenan or IL-6) followed by PGE2 injection into the same muscle	Long duration of hyperalgesia may indicate differential processing of muscular or cutaneous pain by peripheral or central pathways	Pharmacological and non-pharmacological treatments for FM or comorbidities, as well as changes in the CNS, have not yet been studied in this model
Yokoyama et al. [38]	Fatigue-enhanced muscle pain	Running wheel for 2 h followed by two injections of acid saline (pH 5)	Muscle fatigue may increase hyperalgesia produced by low-intensity agents	Pharmacological and non-pharmacological treatments for FM or comorbidities have not yet been determined
Nagakura et al. [39]	Biogenic amine depletion model	Repeated administration of reserpine (1 mg/kg/day, for 3 consecutive days; sc)	Animals show signs of comorbidities as depression and anxiety	It is unclear how changes in the serotonergic system contribute to the maintenance of hyperalgesia. All studies so far have been performed only on males. It is not known if there are differences between males and females
Nishiyori et al. [40]	Cold stress model	Maintenance in cold room (−3 to +4°C) overnight for 3 days and transfer between normal room temperature (24°C) and a cold room every 30 min during the day	Pharmacological treatments directed to FM also have an effect in this model, with the exception of opioids, which are not effective in FM and reduce hyperalgesia in the model cited	Comorbidities such as anxiety and depression are not developed
Khasar et al. [41]	Sound stress model	Exposure to pure tones of 5, 11, 15, and 19 kHz, with amplitudes between 20 and 110 dB in random times each minute, lasting from 5 to 10 s, on days 1, 3, and 4	Anxiety is developed as comorbidity	All studies so far have been performed only on males. It is not known if there are differences between males and females

Note: CNS, central nervous system; FM, fibromyalgia.

Table 1. Summary of major animal models of fibromyalgia.

http://dx.doi.org/10.5772/intechopen.70016

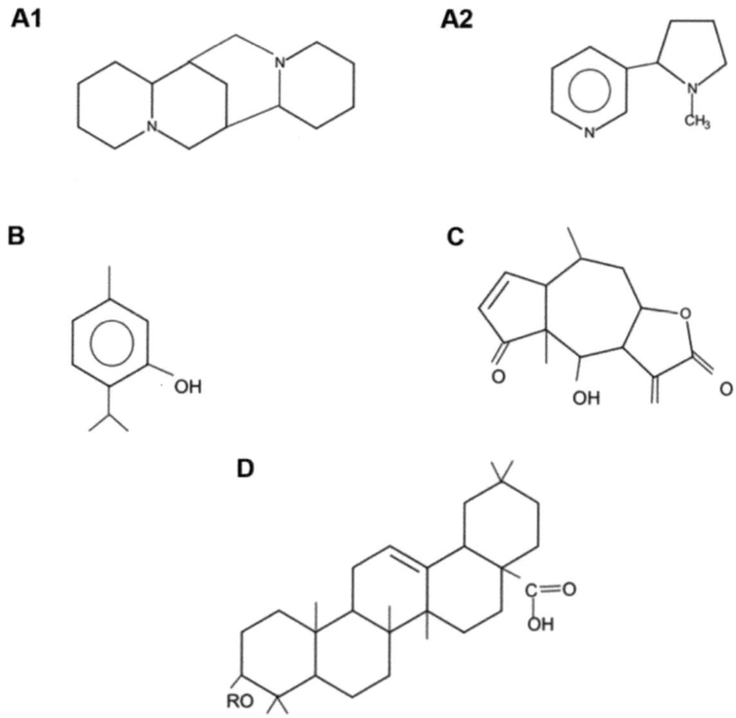

Figure 1. General structures of different categories of bioactive plant compounds studied for the treatment of FM: alkaloids (A1 and A2); monoterpenes (B); sesquiterpenes (C); and triterpenes, saponins, and steroids (D) (adapted from Azmir et al. [42]).

Natural product	Dose/route	Type of study	Sample	Molecular mechanism	References
Essential oils					
Hyptis pectinata	0.3 ml/mouse (5%); sc	Preclinical	Male Swiss mice (n = 8/group)	Opioid, serotoninergic, cholinergic, and reduction of SP, with involvement in the descending pain pathway	Quintans-Júnior et al. [24]
Ocimum basilicum	25, 50, and 100 mg/kg; po	Preclinical	Male Swiss mice (n = 8/group)	Opioid, glutamatergic, TRPV1, and reduction of SP, with involvement in the descending pain pathway	Nascimento et al. [25]
O24™	Not described; to	Clinical	133 subjects of either sex	Stimulation of A-beta sensory fibers and inhibition of bradykinin, histamine, and prostaglandins	Ko et al. [26]

Natural product	Dose/route	Type of study	Sample	Molecular mechanism	References
Plant extracts					
Phyllanthus amarus and *Phyllanthus fraternus*	400 mg/kg; ip	Preclinical	Male Wistar rats (n = 5/group)	Opioid	Chopade and Sayyad [27]
Ginkgo biloba	200 mg/day; po	Clinical	25 subjects of either sex	Antioxidant	Lister et al. [28]
Terpenes					
Linalool	25 mg/kg; po	Preclinical	Male Swiss mice (n = 8/group)	Opioid, glutamatergic, and blocking of neuronal excitability	Nascimento et al. [29]
Citronellal	50 mg/kg; po	Preclinical	Male Swiss mice (n = 7/group)	Opioid, glutamatergic, SP pathway, TRPV1 receptor, involvement in the descending pain pathway, and blocking of sodium channels	Santos et al. [30]
α-Terpineol	25, 50, and 100 mg/kg; po	Preclinical	Male Swiss mice (n = 8/group)	Opioid, serotoninergic, glutamatergic, TRPV1, and reduction of SP, with involvement in the descending pain pathway	Oliveira et al. [31]
β-Caryophyllene	10 and 20 mg/kg; po	Preclinical	Male Swiss mice (n = 8/group)	Opioid and cannabinoid	Quintans-Júnior et al. [32]
Saponin					
Hecogenin acetate	20 mg/kg; po	Preclinical	Male Swiss mice (n = 8/group)	Opioid, SP, ATP-sensitive K (+) channel, with involvement in the descending pain pathway	Quintans et al. [33]
Alkaloid					
Capsaicin	0.075% (3 times/day); to	Clinical	126 women and 4 men	TRPV1 and reduction of SP	Casanueva et al. [34]

*All preclinical studies used the chronic muscle pain model induced by acid saline.

Note: ATP, adenosine triphosphate; ip, intraperitoneal; po, oral administration; sc, subcutaneous; SP, substance P; to, topically; TRPV1, transient receptor potential vanilloid 1.

Table 2. Summary of studies involving bioatctive compounds aimed at the treatment of fibromyalgia and their main mechanisms of action.

2. Pharmacology of bioactive compounds

Bioactive compounds, produced by plants, are designated secondary metabolites. Metabolites can be divided into primary and secondary. Primary metabolites are those involved in growth and development, such as carbohydrates, amino acids, proteins, and lipids, while secondary metabolites, which often have unusual chemical structures, are not required for primary metabolic processes and are believed to support plant survival with respect to local challenges. Thus, the production of secondary metabolites of a given species will be related to their need for survival. Among the secondary metabolites, some compounds have an effect on biological systems, being considered bioactive, which defines them as secondary metabolites of plants that induce pharmacological or toxic effects in humans or animals [42].

Bioactive compounds can be extracted from various parts of the plant, such as the leaves, seeds, flowers, bark, roots, and fruits [43]. These compounds form the essential oil of the plant, resin, or other plant products, which can be extracted in a concentrated form (containing secondary metabolites) or by means of solvents, such as water, ethanol, methanol, chloroform, dichloromethane, ether, and acetone [42]. The best solvent or extraction procedure will depend on the botanical material to be used as well as of the type of secondary metabolites being obtained. In addition, various substances can be isolated from the essential oil or chemical extracts, such as terpenes, flavonoids, alkaloid, and steroids that already have some known property that can be used in the treatment of FM [43].

2.1. Essential oils

Essential oils (EOs) are derived from the secondary metabolism of aromatic plants and are mainly terpene compounds. They are volatile and usually have a strong and characteristic smell. In nature, they perform plant protection functions against predators and help attract certain animals for pollination. In industry, they are used for numerous purposes including in perfume, as antiseptics, and food preservatives but also have numerous pharmacological properties [44]. They are mixtures and may contain 20–60 compounds (or more) in varying concentrations. Usually, each EO is characterized by its major components, which may be number two or three and usually be between 20 and 70% of the oil [45].

Although the biological effect of EOs are thought to be due to the major components which define their pharmacological profiles, synergism between the molecules present in each oil, even those that are in a smaller quantity, can modulate the effects of the major components [45].

2.2. Plant extracts

Based on non-pharmacological studies and holistic or alternative medicine with the use of medicinal plants (and related products), several researchers have sought to evaluate the effects of materials obtained through NPs in clinical and preclinical studies. This research has been based on the popular and potentially dangerous belief given the chemical diversity of NPs that "what is natural, cannot do you harm." The innovative pharmacological effects that these products are able to produce are promising but due to possible side effects remain challenging at the same time [50–52]. One way to evaluate possible pharmacological effects and examine their use in folk medicine is to study plant extracts obtained through the use of several solvents [53–55]. The extraction of biological products using solvents is mainly used with fragile or delicate flower materials, which do not tolerate the heat of steam distillation. Examples of solvents which may be used to produce plant extracts are acetone, hexane, ether, methanol, or ethanol [43]. These extracts, in turn, can have a limited use due to their high viscosity, facilitating aggregation and precipitation, or the presence of proteins that induce false results, causing better ways of obtaining and fractionating the crude extracts to be sought [54].

2.3. Terpenes

Terpenes are the largest group of secondary metabolites obtained through natural products, being made from isoprene units (five carbons (C5)). They exhibit a wide variety of structures and are the most common class of chemical compounds found in essential oils [43, 46–48]. Essential oils contain mainly monoterpenes (C10) and sesquiterpenes (C15), which are generally hydrocarbons of the general formula (C5H8)n. At a lower concentration, they are present in essential oils as diterpenes (C20), triterpenes (C30), and tetraterpenes (C40), which are larger molecules. Terpenoids are oxygen compounds that can be derived from terpenes. These compounds may present predominantly as phenols, monoterpene alcohol, sesquiterpene alcohol, aldehydes, ketones, esters, oxides, lactones, and ethers [43].

Although monoterpenes are smaller molecules than sesquiterpenes, the structure and functional properties of these groups are similar [43, 49]. Most monoterpenes are colorless, volatile, and lipophilic, which promote greater penetration through the membrane [49]. Among the activities already described, the antinociceptive properties of these compounds have received a lot of attention [50–52].

2.4. Saponin

Triterpenoid or steroidal aglycones linked to portions of oligosaccharides are called saponins. Saponins are amphipathic because of the combination of the aglycone, having hydrophobic characteristics, and sugar molecules, with a hydrophilic profile. These compounds have been studied for use in the pharmaceutical, cosmetic, agronomic, and food industries [53]. Saponins present some therapeutic activities including powerful membrane-permeabilizing agents with hypocholesterolemic, immunostimulatory, anti-inflammatory, antimicrobial, anticarcinogenic, antiprotozoan, molluscicides, and antioxidant properties [54]. The majority of plant species-producing saponins are dicotyledonous and accumulate mainly triterpenoid saponins. The monocotyledon type mainly synthesizes saponins of the steroidal type [55].

2.5. Alkaloids

Alkaloids are complex compounds that contain nitrogen. These compounds have been used in the production of various drugs, such as metronidazole (derived from azomycin) and bedaquiline (derived from quinolone) [56–60]. Capsaicin is an alkaloid derived from hot chili peppers from the *Capsicum*. This alkaloid interacts with afferent nociceptors by means of the vanilloid receptors, resulting in increased sensitivity, which is perceived as pruritus, stinging, or burning. This happens due to selective activation of type C afferent fibers, release of substance P, and cutaneous vasodilation. Capsaicin-based topical creams have been used in the treatment of painful disorders such as musculoskeletal or neuropathic disorders, probably functioning by depletion of substance P in the afferent nerve endings [34, 61–63].

3. Preclinical studies

Recently, Quintans-Júnior et al. [24] evaluated pretreatment with the EO from *Hyptis pectinata* loaded in a nanoemulsion thermoreversible gel in an animal model of noninflammatory chronic muscular pain, an experimental model for FM. This pharmaceutical formulation containing EO and Pluronic F127-based hydrogel produced a long-lasting and consistent anti-hyperalgesic effect for 10 days after a single subcutaneous application, which was reversed by naloxone (opioid antagonist) and methysergide (serotoninergic antagonist). In addition, the formulation produced a significant reduction in substance P (SP) levels in the spinal cord. Moreover, it was also shown to increase neuron activation, by Fos protein expression, in the periaqueductal gray (PAG), the nucleus raphe magnus (NRM), and the locus coeruleus (LC), the CNS areas reported to be involved in the descending pathway of pain, so it appears that the formulation acts by improving the endogenous analgesia mechanism (**Figure 3**). Other studies have demonstrated that *H. pectinata* essential oil exhibits antinociceptive effects, probably mediated by the opioid and cholinergic receptors [64, 65].

Nascimento et al. [25] demonstrated in the same FM animal model that *Ocimum basilicum* essential oil, rich in monoterpenes such as linalool, has an important anti-hyperalgesic profile when complexed or noncomplexed with β-cyclodextrin (β-CD). Moreover, the complexed oil produced a long-lasting anti-hyperalgesic effect when compared to the oil alone, demonstrating that the complexation process allows greater stability and bioavailability of the oil or its main compounds, such as monoterpenes. In this paper, the authors also assessed Fos protein expression in the brains of mice and found that this oil promoted the activation of the PAG, NRM, and LC, which are encephalic regions that participate in the antinociceptive effect by the activation of the pain inhibitory descending pathway.

The results obtained for the *O. basilicum* essential oil may be due to its action on the inhibition of SP or through blocking the neurokinin-1 receptor and the vanilloid receptor (TRPV1). Indeed, this oil also acts by glutamatergic system inhibition or by the inhibition of inflammatory pathways, because it was able to produce a reduction in orofacial nociception when caused by formalin, capsaicin, and glutamate in mice [66]. Furthermore, when assessed using an electrophysiological approach, this oil was able to inhibit an orthodromic response in the dentate hippocampal gyrus, similar to DNQX (a glutamatergic drug), an AMPA and kainate receptor antagonist. In addition, another study carried out by Venâncio et al. [67] demonstrated that the peripheral and central antinociceptive effects of *O. basilicum* essential oil are related to the inhibition of the biosynthesis of pain mediators, such as prostaglandins and prostacyclins, and its ability to interact with opioid receptors.

Some studies using plant extracts for the treatment of FM have been performed. Chopade and Sayyad [27] used aqueous, methanolic, hydromethanolic, and hydroethanolic extracts of the genus *Phyllanthus* in an animal model of FM induced by acid saline. It was observed that the extract was able to reduce hyperalgesia without causing tolerance. Extracts of these plants have shown an antinociceptive effect, including in the hot-plate test [68]. In addition, there are indications these extracts depressed the CNS without apparently causing nervous toxicity or altering motor coordination, which may have corroborated with the anti-hyperalgesic effect obtained in the FM animal model [69].

The variability of the pharmacological mechanisms of terpenes and related compounds is shown in **Figure 2**, especially when incorporated into pharmaceutical formulations which improve their pharmacological properties. Moreover, β-caryophyllene, a major compound of *H. pectinata* leaf essential oil (HpEO), complexed with β-cyclodextrin decreased Fos protein expression in the superficial dorsal horn, which seems to involve the descending inhibitory pain system in an animal model of FM (**Figure 2(C)**). Germacrene D, another major component

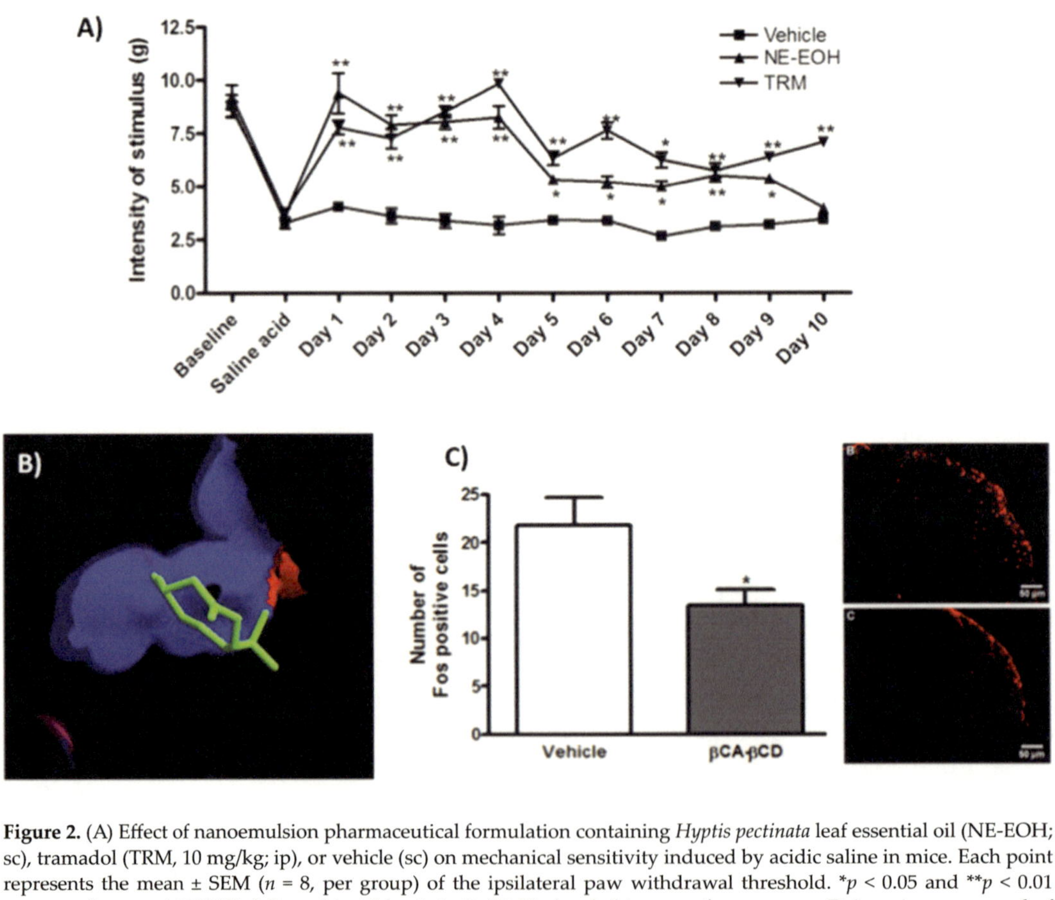

Figure 2. (A) Effect of nanoemulsion pharmaceutical formulation containing *Hyptis pectinata* leaf essential oil (NE-EOH; sc), tramadol (TRM, 10 mg/kg; ip), or vehicle (sc) on mechanical sensitivity induced by acidic saline in mice. Each point represents the mean ± SEM (n = 8, per group) of the ipsilateral paw withdrawal threshold. *$p < 0.05$ and **$p < 0.01$ vs. control group (ANOVA followed by Tukey's test). (B) Hydrophobic map of germacrene D (a major compound of *Hyptis pectinata* leaf essential oil) and μ-opioid receptor (μ-OR). Blue, hydrophobic region; red, hydrophilic region. (C) Fos-positive neurons in the lumbar spinal cord lamina I. Vehicle or β-caryophyllene-β-cyclodextrin (20 mg/kg) was administered orally, and, after 90 min, the animals were perfused (adapted from Quintans-Júnior et al. [25, 33]).

http://dx.doi.org/10.5772/intechopen.70016

of HpEO, has a strong interaction with the μ-opioid receptor (**Figure 2(B)**). A more interesting aspect was that when the HpEO was incorporated in a nanoemulsion thermoreversible pluronic F127-based hydrogel, it produced a long-lasting and consistent anti-hyperalgesic effect (**Figure 2(A)**), suggesting that essential oils and their major components are promising tools for managing FM.

Some studies involving the effects of monoterpenes in FM experimental models have been undertaken due to their possible molecular effects on pain (**Figure 3**) [52]. Nascimento et al. [29] used linalool (**Figure 4**), a monoterpene present in plant species of the family Lamiaceae, complexed and noncomplexed in β-CD, in an animal model of FM and observed that both

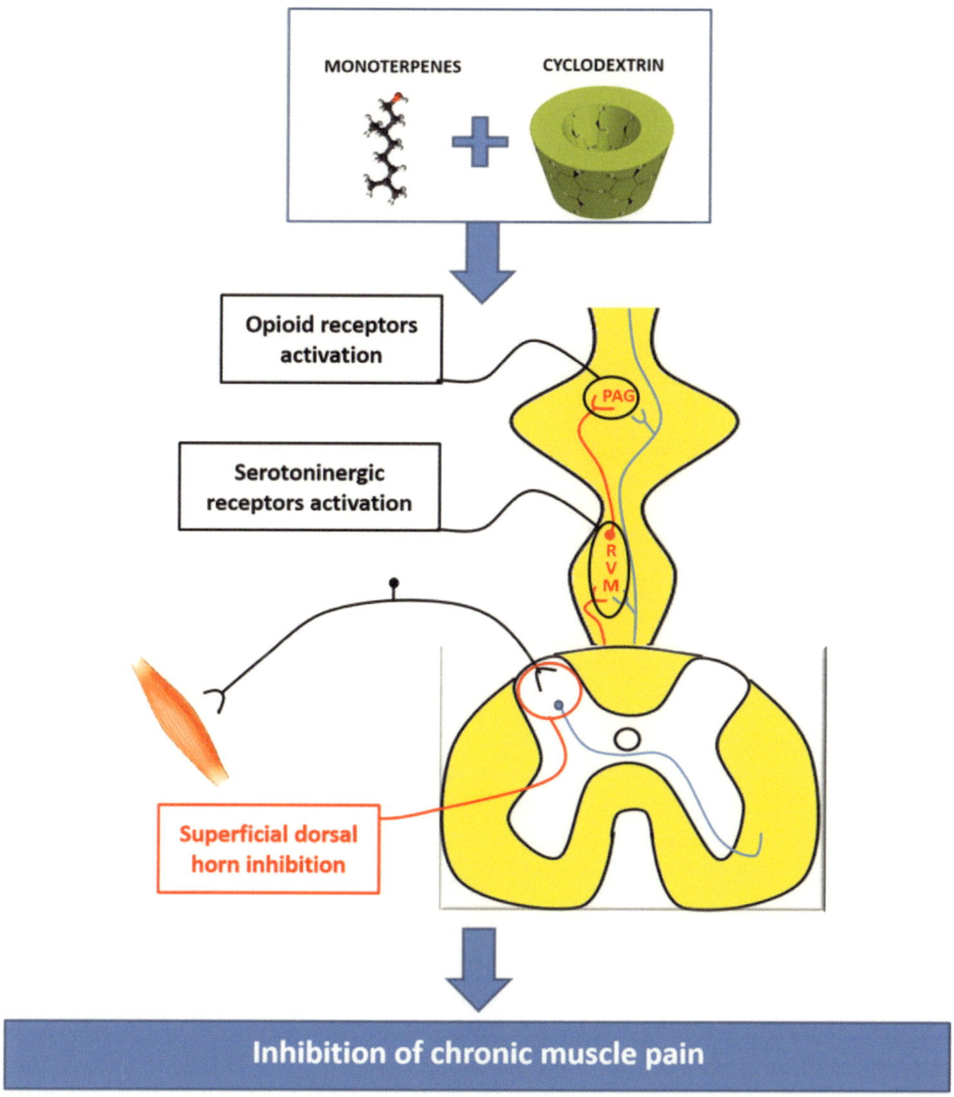

Figure 3. Schematic illustration of descending pain pathway and cyclodextrin complexation with monoterpenes (adapted from Quintans-Júnior et al. [24]).

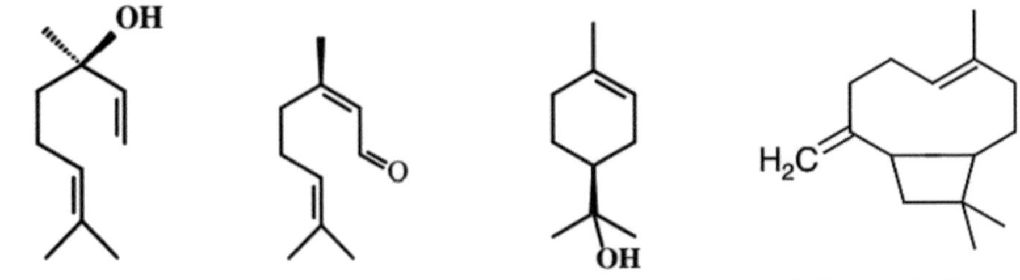

Figure 4. Structure of terpenes studied for the treatment of FM (adapted from Guimarães et al. [23, 52]).

formulations had an anti-hyperalgesic effect, with the complexed form being more effective and producing a longer-lasting effect (for 24 h after administration). Previous studies have shown the analgesic effect of linalool on acute central nociception (hot plate), visceral (acetic acid) [70] and chronic pain models of neuropathic origin [71, 72], and the opioid and glutamatergic systems probably being involved in this action [73]. Moreover, linalool was able to reduce the action potential amplitude assessed using an isolated nerve in the single sucrose-gap technique, showing it blocked neuronal excitability [74].

The possible benefits of the complexation of apolar compounds (such as terpenes) with CDs have been explored by the pharmaceutical industry and by researchers seeking improvements in pharmacological properties such as increased bioavailability, efficacy, and optimization of therapeutic doses (which reduces toxicity and adverse effects) [75, 76]. Clinical and preclinical evidence has shown that the pharmacological effects of analgesic and anti-inflammatory drugs are improved when complexed with CDs [76–78].

Santos et al. [30] evaluated the effect of citronellal (**Figure 4**), a monoterpene present in *Citrus* and *Cymbopogon* plants, complexed in β-CD as a potential agent against FM symptoms. It was observed that complexation in CD improved the anti-hyperalgesic effect when compared to noncomplexed citronellal. This effect probably involves activation of descending pain pathway areas, such as the PAG and rostroventromedial (RVM) areas, with possible interaction with the glutamate receptors, investigated by a docking study. Citronellal has already presented an antinociceptive effect on capsaicin, glutamate, and formalin-induced orofacial pain, showing that this terpene may be acting via SP and TRPV1 receptors or in the glutamatergic pathway [79]. In addition, the analgesic effect of citronellal was reversed by naloxone in hot-plate tests, which strongly suggests its action on the opioid receptors and its ability to reduce neuronal excitability through blocking sodium channels [51, 79].

Another study, also using the chronic noninflammatory widespread pain model in mice (an FM animal model), evaluated the effect of α-terpineol (**Figure 4**), both pure and complexed in β-CD, as CDs are useful tools in improving the pharmacological properties of terpenes [77, 80]. The authors observed an anti-hyperalgesic effect, possibly related to the action of α-terpineol on the opioid and serotonergic receptors; visualized with the use of naloxone and ondansetron antagonists; and confirmed by docking studies [31]. Similarly to citronellal, α-terpineol also showed antinociceptive effect in the capsaicin, glutamate, and formalin-induced orofacial nociception tests [81], indicating other possible mechanisms of action of this monoterpene. In summary, it has been shown that monoterpenes complexed in β-cyclodextrin reduce hyperalgesia induced by chronic muscle pain, activating the descending pathway, as described in **Figure 3**.

Sesquiterpenes occur *in nature* as hydrocarbons or in oxygenated forms including lactones, alcohols, acids, aldehydes, and ketones. Biosynthesis of sesquiterpenes can occur by the mevalonic acid and the deoxyxylulose phosphate pathway. These compounds have various pharmacological activities including antileishmanial, antimalarial, antifungal, antibacterial, antiviral, anti-inflammatory, and antinociceptive properties and the ability to inhibit the production of nitric oxide and eliminate hydroxyl radicals [82].

β-Caryophyllene (**Figure 4**) is a bicyclic sesquiterpene compound found in the EO of the *Eugenia caryophyllata* (cloves) and *Piper nigrum* (black pepper) plant species. In an experimental study conducted in an FM model in mice, this compound, complexed in β-CD, reduced primary and secondary hyperalgesia as well as inhibited the superficial dorsal horn of the spinal cord, possibly by activation of descending pain pathway [32]. Antagonism studies, in a capsaicin-induced nociception test, showed that the antinociceptive effect of β-caryophyllene was reversed by naloxone, β-funaltrexamine (a μ-opioid receptor antagonist), and AM630 (a CB2 receptor antagonist) [83]. In addition, in a neuropathic pain model, β-caryophyllene had an effect on thermal hyperalgesia and mechanical allodynia, reducing spinal neuroinflammation. The oral administration of β-caryophyllene was more effective than the subcutaneously injected synthetic CB2 agonist JWH-133 [84].

Quintans et al. [33] evaluated the effect of hecogenin acetate (HA), an acetylated steroidal saponin, complexed with β-CD in a chronic noninflammatory widespread pain model. Hecogenin is already used in the pharmaceutical industry to synthesize some oral contraceptive agents. The effect of noncomplexed or complexed HA caused an increase in the nociceptive threshold and primary and secondary hyperalgesia compared to the vehicle control group. However, the HA/β-CD complex was superior in producing an analgesic profile using lower nominal doses of the active principle (HA). In addition, the interaction of the HA with opioid receptors and a decrease in SP levels in the lumbar spinal cord were verified, which indicate participation of this substance in the descending inhibitory pain pathway [33, 85].

The antinociceptive effect of HA was previously observed in the tail-flick test. This effect was reversed by naloxone, CTOP (μ-opioid receptor antagonist), nor-BNI (κ-opioid receptor antagonist), naltrindole (δ-opioid receptor antagonist), and glibenclamide (ATP-sensitive K (+) channel blocker). Mice pretreated with HA had increased neuronal activation in the PAG area, suggesting the participation of the endogenous analgesia pathway in the hecogenin mechanism of action [85].

Some clinical studies with EOs have been developed in humans with FM. O24™ is a blend of six essential oils: aloe vera, eucalyptus, lemon/orange, camphor, rosemary, and peppermint. This mixture is marketed for the relief of pain. In a double-blinded randomized clinical trial, Ko et al. [26] demonstrated the benefits of using this oil, topically, for FM pain relief. Males and females were recruited for the study through newspapers and internet communications.

FM diagnosis was confirmed before the patients enrolled in the study. The authors reveal that the main mode of action is as a counterirritant to the pain sensation. The mixture of oils promotes stimulation of A-beta sensory fibers, causing inhibition of the A-delta and C fibers. Moreover, the local effects of O24™ include the inhibition of bradykinin, histamine, and prostaglandins, which do not seem to be directly related to the analgesic effect in FM, so it is more reasonable to propose its effect indirectly in the pathways of pain modulation.

Rutledge and Jones [86] also investigated the topical effect of O24 in a double-blind randomized clinical trial associated with exercises multilevel for 12 weeks. Twenty patients with FM and 23 patients of the sham group were submitted to the study. There was no statistical difference between the groups regarding the pain and physical function, but there was improvement of the physical function, without statistical difference, when compared before and after the treatment, keeping the effect of O24 on the FM symptoms unknown. This result for O24 differs from that described by Ko et al. [26], which may result from the small sample and the type of exercise used, since some exercises may contribute to the maintenance of pain in patients with FM [3].

The effect of *Ginkgo biloba* extract and the coenzyme Q10 was evaluated in 23 fibromyalgic patients, before and after the treatment, by oral administration, for 12 weeks, with 64% of patients reporting an improvement in quality of life through the application of questionnaires. The improvement observed by these patients may be related in parts to the antioxidant activities described for both coenzyme Q10 and *Ginkgo biloba* [28].

Due to the properties attributed to capsaicin, Casanueva et al. [34] evaluated the short-term efficacy of topical capsaicin treatment in 130 patients with fibromyalgia who were already using drug therapy. Patients were randomly divided into a control group (same medical treatment that they received before randomization) and topical capsaicin group (medical treatment that they received before randomization + 0.075% capsaicin) by a computer-generated sequence. After 6 weeks, it was observed that the additional topical treatment reduced the myalgia score and improved the quality of life of these patients, showing that capsaicin was also effective in this syndrome.

4. Final considerations

Fibromyalgia is the second most common rheumatologic disorder, being characterized by the manifestation of widespread pain with sensory changes. The treatment strategies for the management of the FM include both pharmacological products (such as duloxetine, pregabalina, and tramadol for pain and amitriptyline, cyclobenzaprine, and pregabalina for sleep disturbance) and non-pharmacological therapies (such as exercise and psychological therapies) [87]. Despite this, fibromyalgia remains difficult to treat and is an important challenge for modern medicine, as the treatments for these conditions are still ineffective with a large number of side effects, making the search for new treatments ever more urgent.

In this context, one important approach to the discovery of new medicines with analgesic activity is research with natural products. For thousands of years, scientists and the pharmaceutical industry have used natural products as a source for new drugs or their

http://dx.doi.org/10.5772/intechopen.70016

precursors, aimed at treating diseases or symptomatology that had no effective treatment. Despite of the animal models described for FM, some limitations can be observed, such as the reversion of the pain with opioid treatment and the absence of other signs and symptoms observed in humans. However, these models are the most resembled FM in humans, being tools used in the search for new treatment options. Nowadays, many natural substances have been studied, clinically and preclinically, for their analgesic potential with respect to fibromyalgia. In this context, essential oils, plant extracts, terpenes, and alkaloids are major sources of natural products.

These substances have been shown to have an analgesic effect in animal models of fibromyalgia, acting through different pathways, including activation of the descending inhibitory pain pathway—specifically the opioid, glutamatergic, cannabinoid, and serotoninergic systems; inhibition of SP in the superficial dorsal horn of the spinal cord; blockage of peripheral fibers; and antioxidant activity. In addition, clinical studies have shown the importance of NPs in the pain management of FM, improving their quality of life. The effective use of these products in the clinic, without reports of considerable adverse effects, describes the advances in the use of NPs in the treatment of FM. These finding make natural products a promising source of treatments for the management of chronic pain.

Acknowledgements

This work was supported by grants from CNPq (305608/2013-4, 311721/2014-1), CAPES, and FAPITEC/SE (Chamadas Públicas PROMOB e PROEF), all from Brazil. PL Santos, RG Brito, and MA Oliveira were carrying out the master's or PhD degrees in the Graduate Program in Health Sciences (PPGCS/UFS), and LTS Pina was carrying out the master's degree in the Graduate Program in Pharmaceutical Sciences (PPGCF/UFS).

Author details

Renan Guedes Brito[1], Priscila Laise Santos[1], Marlange Almeida Oliveira[1], Lícia Tairiny Santos Pina[1], Angelo Roberto Antoniolli[1], Jackson Roberto Guedes da Silva Almeida[2], Laurent Picot[3], Gokhan Zengin[4], Jullyana Souza Siqueira Quintans[1] and Lucindo José Quintans Júnior[1*]

*Address all correspondence to: lucindojr@gmail.com

1 Laboratory of Neuroscience and Pharmacological Assays (LANEF), Department of Physiology, Federal University of Sergipe (UFS), São Cristóvão, SE, Brazil

2 Center for Studies and Research of Medicinal Plants, Federal University of San Francisco Valley, Petrolina, Pernambuco, Brazil

3 Faculty of Science and Technology, University of La Rochelle, La Rochelle, France

4 Department of Biology, Science Faculty, Selcuk University, Konya, Turkey

References

[1] Gauffin J, Hankama T, Kautiainen H, Hannonen P, Haanpää M. Neuropathic pain and use of PainDETECT in patients with fibromyalgia: A cohort study. BMC Neurology. 2013 Jan;**13**:21

[2] Bäckryd E, Tanum L, Lind A-L, Larsson A, Gordh T. Evidence of both systemic inflammation and neuroinflammation in fibromyalgia patients, as assessed by a multiplex protein panel applied to the cerebrospinal fluid and to plasma. Journal of Pain Research. 2017 Mar;**10**:515-525

[3] Elvin A, Siösteen A-K, Nilsson A, Kosek E. Decreased muscle blood flow in fibromyalgia patients during standardised muscle exercise: A contrast media enhanced colour Doppler study. European Journal of Pain. 2006 Feb;**10**(2):137-144

[4] Calvino B, Grilo RM. Central pain control. Joint, Bone, Spine. 2006 Jan;**73**(1):10-16

[5] Perl ER. Pain mechanisms: A commentary on concepts and issues. Progress in Neurobiology. 2011 Jun;**94**(1):20-38

[6] Clauw DJ, Arnold LM, McCarberg BH, FibroCollaborative. The science of fibromyalgia. Mayo Clinic Proceedings. 2011 Sep;**86**(9):907-911

[7] Merskey H, Bogduk N. Classification of Chronic Pain: Descriptions of Chronic Pain Syndromes and Definitions of Pain Terms. 2nd ed. Seatle: IASP; 1994. 240 p

[8] Mist SD, Firestone KA, Jones KD. Complementary and alternative exercise for fibromyalgia: A meta-analysis. Journal of Pain Research. 2013 Jan;**6**:247-260

[9] Crofford LJ, Rowbotham MC, Mease PJ, Russell IJ, Dworkin RH, Corbin AE, et al. Pregabalin for the treatment of fibromyalgia syndrome: Results of a randomized, double-blind, placebo-controlled trial. Arthritis and Rheumatism. 2005 Apr;**52**(4):1264-1273

[10] Mease PJ, Dundon K, Sarzi-Puttini P. Pharmacotherapy of fibromyalgia. Best Practice & Research. Clinical Rheumatology. 2011 Apr;**25**(2):285-297

[11] Häuser W, Petzke F, Sommer C. Comparative efficacy and harms of duloxetine, milnacipran, and pregabalin in fibromyalgia syndrome. The Journal of Pain. 2010 Jun;**11**(6):505-521

[12] Rehm SE, Koroschetz J, Gockel U, Brosz M, Freynhagen R, Tolle TR, et al. A cross-sectional survey of 3035 patients with fibromyalgia: Subgroups of patients with typical comorbidities and sensory symptom profiles. Rheumatology. 2010 Jun 1;**49**(6):1146-1152

[13] DeSantana JM, da Cruz KML, Sluka KA. Animal models of fibromyalgia. Arthritis Research & Therapy. 2013;**15**(6):222

[14] Mogil JS. Animal models of pain: Progress and challenges. Nature Reviews Neuroscience. 2009 Apr;**10**(4):283-294

[15] Nagakura Y. Recent advancements in animal models of fibromyalgia. MYOPAIN. 2017 Jan **11**;1-8

[16] Sluka KA. Is it possible to develop an animal model of fibromyalgia? Pain. 2009 Nov;**146**(1-2):3-4

[17] Harvey AL, Edrada-Ebel R, Quinn RJ. The re-emergence of natural products for drug discovery in the genomics era. Nature Reviews Drug Discovery. 2015 Jan 23;**14**(2):111-129

[18] Dias DA, Urban S, Roessner U. A historical overview of natural products in drug discovery. Metabolites. 2012 Jan;**2**(2):303-336

[19] Kinghorn AD, Pan L, Fletcher JN, Chai H. The relevance of higher plants in lead compound discovery programs. Journal of Natural Products. 2011 Jun 24;**74**(6):1539-1555

[20] Vane JR. Inhibition of prostaglandin synthesis as a mechanism of action for aspirin-like drugs. Nature. 1971 Jun 23;**231**(25):232-235

[21] Goerig M, Schulte am Esch J. [Friedrich Wilhelm Adam Sertürner—the discoverer of morphine]. Anästhesiologie, Intensivmedizin, Notfallmedizin, Schmerztherapie. 1991 Dec;**26**(8):492-498

[22] McCurdy CR, Scully SS. Analgesic substances derived from natural products (natureceuticals). Life Sciences. 2005 Dec 22;**78**(5):476-484

[23] Guimarães AG, Serafini MR, Quintans-Júnior LJ. Terpenes and derivatives as a new perspective for pain treatment: A patent review. Expert Opinion on Therapeutic Patents. 2014 Mar;**24**(3):243-265

[24] Quintans-Júnior LJ, Brito RG, Quintans JSS, Santos PL, Camargo ZT, Barreto PA, et al. Nanoemulsion thermoreversible pluronic F127-based hydrogel containing *Hyptis pectinata* (Lamiaceae) leaf essential oil produced a lasting anti-hyperalgesic effect in chronic noninflammatory widespread pain in mice. Molecular Neurobiology. 2017 Feb 13

[25] Nascimento SS, Araújo AAS, Brito RG, Serafini MR, Menezes PP, DeSantana JM, et al. Cyclodextrin-complexed *Ocimum basilicum* leaves essential oil increases Fos protein expression in the central nervous system and produce an antihyperalgesic effect in animal models for fibromyalgia. International Journal of Molecular Sciences. 2015 Jan;**16**(1):547-563

[26] Ko GD, Hum A, Traitses G, Berbrayer D. Effects of topical O24 essential oils on patients with fibromyalgia syndrome: A randomized, placebo controlled pilot study. Journal of Musculoskeletal Pain. 2007 Jan 16;**15**(1):11-19

[27] Chopade AR, Sayyad FJ. Antifibromyalgic activity of standardized extracts of *Phyllanthus amarus* and *Phyllanthus fraternus* in acidic saline induced chronic muscle pain. Biomedicine and Aging Pathology. 2014 Apr;**4**(2):123-130

[28] Lister R. An open, pilot study to evaluate the potential benefits of coenzyme Q10 combined with *Ginkgo Biloba* extract in fibromyalgia syndrome. The Journal of International Medical Research. 2002 Apr;**30**(2):195-199

[29] Nascimento SS, Camargo EA, DeSantana JM, Araújo AAS, Menezes PP, Lucca-Júnior W, et al. Linalool and linalool complexed in β-cyclodextrin produce anti-hyperalgesic activity and increase Fos protein expression in animal model for fibromyalgia. Naunyn Schmiedebergs Archives of Pharmacology. 2014 Jun 24

[30] Santos PL, Brito RG, Oliveira MA, Quintans JSS, Guimarães AG, Santos MR V, et al. Docking, characterization and investigation of β-cyclodextrin complexed with citronellal, a monoterpene present in the essential oil of Cymbopogon species, as an anti-hyperalgesic agent in chronic muscle pain model. Phytomedicine. 2016 Aug 15;**23**(9):948-957

[31] Oliveira MGB, Brito RG, Santos PL, Araújo-Filho HG, Quintans JSS, Menezes PP, et al. α-Terpineol, a monoterpene alcohol, complexed with β-cyclodextrin exerts antihyperalgesic effect in animal model for fibromyalgia aided with docking study. Chemico-Biological Interactions. 2016 Jul 25;**254**:54-62

[32] Quintans-Júnior LJ, Araújo AAS, Brito RG, Santos PL, Quintans JSS, Menezes PP, et al. β-Caryophyllene, a dietary cannabinoid, complexed with β-cyclodextrin produced anti-hyperalgesic effect involving the inhibition of Fos expression in superficial dorsal horn. Life Sciences. 2016 Mar;**149**:34-41

[33] Quintans JSS, Pereira EWM, Carvalho YMBG, Menezes PP, Serafini MR, Batista MVA, et al. Host-guest inclusion complexation of β-cyclodextrin and hecogenin acetate to enhance anti-hyperalgesic effect in an animal model of musculoskeletal pain. Process Biochemistry. 2016 Aug;**52**:1-15

[34] Casanueva B, Rodero B, Quintial C, Llorca J, González-Gay MA. Short-term efficacy of topical capsaicin therapy in severely affected fibromyalgia patients. Rheumatology International. 2013 Oct 28;**33**(10):2665-2670

[35] Sluka KA, Kalra A, Moore SA. Unilateral intramuscular injections of acidic saline produce a bilateral, long-lasting hyperalgesia. Muscle & Nerve. 2001 Jan;**24**(1):37-46

[36] Dina OA, Levine JD, Green PG. Muscle inflammation induces a protein kinase Cε-dependent chronic-latent muscle pain. The Journal of Pain. 2008 May;**9**(5):457-462

[37] Dina OA, Green PG, Levine JD. Role of interleukin-6 in chronic muscle hyperalgesic priming. Neuroscience. 2008 Mar 18;**152**(2):521-525

[38] Yokoyama T, Lisi TL, Moore SA, Sluka KA. Muscle fatigue increases the probability of developing hyperalgesia in mice. The Journal of Pain. 2007 Sep;**8**(9):692-699

[39] Nagakura Y, Oe T, Aoki T, Matsuoka N. Biogenic amine depletion causes chronic muscular pain and tactile allodynia accompanied by depression: A putative animal model of fibromyalgia. Pain. 2009 Nov;**146**(1):26-33

[40] Nishiyori M, Uchida H, Nagai J, Araki K, Mukae T, Kishioka S, et al. Permanent relief from intermittent cold stress-induced fibromyalgia-like abnormal pain by repeated intrathecal administration of antidepressants. Molecular Pain. 2011 Sep 21;**7**:69

[41] Khasar SG, Dina OA, Green PG, Levine JD. Sound stress-induced long-term enhancement of mechanical hyperalgesia in rats is maintained by sympathoadrenal catecholamines. The Journal of Pain. 2009 Oct;**10**(10):1073-1077

[42] Azmir J, Zaidul ISM, Rahman MM, Sharif KM, Mohamed A, Sahena F, et al. Techniques for extraction of bioactive compounds from plant materials: A review. Journal of Food Engineering. 2013 Aug;**117**(4):426-436

[43] Tongnuanchan P, Benjakul S. Essential oils: Extraction, bioactivities, and their uses for food preservation. Journal of Food Science. 2014 Jul;**79**(7):R1231-R1249

[44] de Souza Nascimento S, Desantana JM, Nampo FK, Ribeiro EAN, da Silva DL, Araújo-Júnior JX, et al. Efficacy and safety of medicinal plants or related natural products for fibromyalgia: A systematic review. Evidence-based Complementary and Alternative Medicine. 2013;**2013**:149468

[45] Bakkali F, Averbeck S, Averbeck D, Idaomar M. Biological effects of essential oils—A review. Food and Chemical Toxicology. 2008 Feb;**46**(2):446-475

[46] Nikolić B, Vasilijević B, Mitić-Ćulafić D, Vuković-Gačić B, Knežević-Vukćević J. Comparative study of genotoxic, antigenotoxic and cytotoxic activities of monoterpenes camphor, eucalyptol and thujone in bacteria and mammalian cells. Chemico-Biological Interactions. 2015 Dec 5;**242**:263-271

[47] Caldas GFR, Limeira MMF, Araújo AV, Albuquerque GS, Silva-Neto JD, Silva TG, et al. Repeated-doses and reproductive toxicity studies of the monoterpene 1,8-cineole (eucalyptol) in Wistar rats. Food and Chemical Toxicology. 2016 Nov;**97**:297-306

[48] Gautam LN, Ling T, Lang W, Rivas F. Anti-proliferative evaluation of monoterpene derivatives against leukemia. European Journal of Medicinal Chemistry. 2016 May 4;**113**:75-80

[49] Oz M, Lozon Y, Sultan A, Yang K-HS, Galadari S. Effects of monoterpenes on ion channels of excitable cells. Pharmacology & Therapeutics. 2015 Aug;**152**:83-97

[50] Brito RG, Guimarães AG, Quintans JSS, Santos MRV, De Sousa DP, Badaue-Passos D, et al. Citronellol, a monoterpene alcohol, reduces nociceptive and inflammatory activities in rodents. Journal of Natural Medicines. 2012 Oct;**66**(4):637-644

[51] Melo MS, Sena LCS, Barreto FJN, Bonjardim LR, Almeida JRGS, Lima JT, et al. Antinociceptive effect of citronellal in mice. Pharmaceutical Biology. 2010 Apr;**48**(4): 411-416

[52] Guimarães AG, Quintans JSS, Quintans LJJ. Monoterpenes with analgesic activity—A systematic review. Phytherapy Research PTR. 2013 Jan;**27**(1):1-15

[53] Dixon RA, Pasinetti GM. Flavonoids and isoflavonoids: From plant biology to agriculture and neuroscience. Plant Physiology. 2010 Oct 1;**154**(2):453-457

[54] Moses T, Papadopoulou KK, Osbourn A. Metabolic and functional diversity of saponins, biosynthetic intermediates and semi-synthetic derivatives. Critical Reviews in Biochemistry and Molecular Biology. 2014 Nov 6;**49**(6):439-462

[55] Sparg SG, Light ME, van Staden J. Biological activities and distribution of plant saponins. Journal of Ethnopharmacology. 2004 Oct;**94**(2-3):219-243

[56] Cushnie TPT, Cushnie B, Lamb AJ. Alkaloids: An overview of their antibacterial, antibiotic-enhancing and antivirulence activities. International Journal of Antimicrobial Agents. 2014 Nov;**44**(5):377-386

[57] Hesse M. Alkaloids : Nature's Curse or Blessing? Verlag Helvetica Chimica Acta; 2002. 413 p

[58] Hraiech S, Bregeon F, Brunel J-M, Rolain J-M, Lepidi H, Andrieu V, et al. Antibacterial efficacy of inhaled squalamine in a rat model of chronic *Pseudomonas aeruginosa* pneumonia. The Journal of Antimicrobial Chemotherapy. 2012 Oct 1;**67**(10):2452-2458

[59] Bogatcheva E, Hanrahan C, Nikonenko B, de los Santos G, Reddy V, Chen P, et al. Identification of SQ609 as a lead compound from a library of dipiperidines. Bioorganic & Medicinal Chemistry Letters. 2011 Sep 15;**21**(18):5353-5357

[60] Parhi A, Kelley C, Kaul M, Pilch DS, LaVoie EJ. Antibacterial activity of substituted 5-methylbenzo[c]phenanthridinium derivatives. Bioorganic & Medicinal Chemistry Letters. 2012 Dec 1;**22**(23):7080-7083

[61] Nolano M, Simone DA, Wendelschafer-Crabb G, Johnson T, Hazen E, Kennedy WR. Topical capsaicin in humans: Parallel loss of epidermal nerve fibers and pain sensation. Pain. 1999 May;**81**(1-2):135-145

[62] Morgenlander JC, Hurwitz BJ, Massey EW. Cabsaicin for the trunent of pain in Guillain-Barré syndrome. Annals of Neurology. 1990 Aug;**28**(2):199

[63] Mason L, Moore RA, Derry S, Edwards JE, McQuay HJ. Systematic review of topical capsaicin for the treatment of chronic pain. BMJ. 2004 Apr 24;**328**(7446):991

[64] Lisboa ACCD, Mello ICM, Nunes RS, Dos Santos MA, Antoniolli AR, Marçal RM, et al. Antinociceptive effect of *Hyptis pectinata* leaves extracts. Fitoterapia. 2006 Sep;**77**(6):439-442

[65] Raymundo LJRP, Guilhon CC, Alviano DS, Matheus ME, Antoniolli AR, Cavalcanti SCH, et al. Characterisation of the anti-inflammatory and antinociceptive activities of the *Hyptis pectinata* (L.) Poit essential oil. Journal of Ethnopharmacology. 2011 Apr 12;**134**(3):725-732

[66] Venâncio AM, Marchioro M, Estavam CS, Melo MS, Santana MT, Onofre ASC, et al. Ocimum basilicum leaf essential oil and (−)-linalool reduce orofacial nociception in rodents: A behavioral and electrophysiological approach. Revista Brasileira Farmacognosia. 2011 Dec;**21**(6):1043-1051

[67] Venâncio AM, Onofre AS, Lira AF, Alves PB, Blank AF, Antoniolli AR, et al. Chemical composition, acute toxicity, and antinociceptive activity of the essential oil of a plant breeding cultivar of basil (*Ocimum basilicum* L.). Planta Medica. 2011 May;**77**(8):825-829

[68] Chopade A, Sayyad F. Analysis of the mechanisms underlying the analgesic effects of the extracts of *Phyllanthus amarus* & *Phyllanthus fraternus*. Asian Journal of Pharmaceutical Research. 2013;**1**(2):34-39

[69] Chopade A, Sayyad F. Toxicity studies and evaluation of *Phyllanthus amarus* and *Phyllanthus fraternus* extracts on the central nervous system and musculoskeletal function. International Journal of Pharmaceutical, Chemistry Science. 2013;**2**:1333-1338

[70] Peana AT, D'Aquila PS, Chessa ML, Moretti MDL, Serra G, Pippia P. (−)-Linalool produces antinociception in two experimental models of pain. European Journal of Pharmacology. 2003 Jan 26;**460**(1):37-41

[71] Batista PA, de Paula Werner MF, Oliveira EC, Burgos L, Pereira P, da Silva Brum LF, et al. The antinociceptive effect of (−)-linalool in models of chronic inflammatory and neuropathic hypersensitivity in mice. The Journal of Pain. 2010 Nov;**11**(11):1222-1229

[72] Berliocchi L, Russo R, Levato A, Fratto V, Bagetta G, Sakurada S, et al. Chapter 17 (−)-linalool attenuates allodynia in neuropathic pain induced by spinal nerve ligation in C57/Bl6 mice. In: International Review of Neurobiology. 2009. pp. 221-235

[73] Batista PA, Werner MF, Oliveira EC, Burgos L, Pereira P, Brum LF, et al. Evidence for the involvement of ionotropic glutamatergic receptors on the antinociceptive effect of (−)-linalool in mice. Neuroscience Letters. 2008 Aug 8;**440**(3):299-303

[74] de Almeida RN, Araújo DAM, Gonçalves JCR, Montenegro FC, de Sousa DP, Leite JR, et al. Rosewood oil induces sedation and inhibits compound action potential in rodents. Journal of Ethnopharmacology. 2009 Jul 30;**124**(3):440-443

[75] Lima PSS, Lucchese AM, Araújo-Filho HG, Menezes PP, Araújo AAS, Quintans-Júnior LJ, et al. Inclusion of terpenes in cyclodextrins: Preparation, characterization and pharmacological approaches. Carbohydrate Polymers 2016 Oct 20;**151**:965-987

[76] Santos PL, Brito RG, Quintans JSS, Araújo AAS, Menezes IRA, Brogden NK, et al. Cyclodextrins as encapsulation agents to improve the anti-inflammatory drugs profile: A systematic review and meta-analysis. Current Pharmaceutical Design. 2017 Jan 26

[77] Brito RG, Araújo AAS, Quintans JSS, Sluka KA, Quintans Júnior LJ. Enhanced analgesic activity by cyclodextrins—A systematic review and meta-analysis. Expert Opinion on Drug Delivery. 2015

[78] Oliveira MGB, Guimarães AG, Araújo AAS, Quintans JSS, Santos MR V, Quintans-Júnior LJ. Cyclodextrins: Improving the therapeutic response of analgesic drugs: A patent review. Expert Opinion on Therapeutic Patents. 2015 Jan;**25**(8):897-907

[79] Quintans-Júnior LJ, Melo MS, De Sousa DP, Araujo AAS, Onofre ACS, Gelain DP, et al. Antinociceptive effects of citronellal in formalin-, capsaicin-, and glutamate-induced orofacial nociception in rodents and its action on nerve excitability. Journal of Orofacial Pain. 2010 Jan;**24**(3):305-312

[80] Lima PSS, Lucchese AM, Araújo-Filho HG, Menezes PP, Araújo AAS, Quintans-Júnior LJ, et al. Inclusion of terpenes in cyclodextrins: Preparation, characterization and pharmacological approaches. Carbohydrate Polymers. 2016;**151**:965-987

[81] Quintans-Júnior LJ, Oliveira MGB, Santana MF, Santana MT, Guimarães AG, Siqueira JS, et al. α-Terpineol reduces nociceptive behavior in mice. Pharmaceutical Biology. 2011 Jun 8;**49**(6):583-586

[82] Awouafack MD, Tane P, Kuete V, Eloff JN. Sesquiterpenes from the medicinal plants of Africa. In: Medicinal Plant Research in Africa. Elsevier; 2013. pp. 33-103

[83] Katsuyama S, Mizoguchi H, Kuwahata H, Komatsu T, Nagaoka K, Nakamura H, et al. Involvement of peripheral cannabinoid and opioid receptors in β-caryophyllene-induced antinociception. European Journal of Pain. 2013 May;**17**(5):664-675

[84] Klauke A-L, Racz I, Pradier B, Markert A, Zimmer AM, Gertsch J, et al. The cannabinoid CB2 receptor-selective phytocannabinoid beta-caryophyllene exerts analgesic effects in mouse models of inflammatory and neuropathic pain. European Neuropsychopharmacology. 2014 Apr;**24**(4):608-620

[85] Gama KB, Quintans JSS, Antoniolli ÂR, Quintans-Júnior LJ, Santana WA, Branco A, et al. Evidence for the involvement of descending pain-inhibitory mechanisms in the antinociceptive effect of Hecogenin Acetate. Journal of Natural Products. 2013 Apr 26;**76**(4):559-563

[86] Rutledge DN, Jones CJ. Effects of topical essential oil on exercise volume after a 12-week exercise program for women with fibromyalgia: A pilot study. Journal of Alternative and Complementary Medicine. 2007 Dec;**13**(10):1099-1106

[87] Ablin J, Fitzcharles M-A, Buskila D, Shir Y, Sommer C, Häuser W. Treatment of fibromyalgia syndrome: Recommendations of recent evidence-based interdisciplinary guidelines with special emphasis on complementary and alternative therapies. Evidence-Based Complementary and Alternative Medicine eCAM. 2013;**2013**:485272

Chapter 5

Recognize Comorbid Fibromyalgia Syndrome in Order to Better Evaluate Selected Rheumatic Diseases

William S. Wilke

Additional information is available at the end of the chapter

http://dx.doi.org/10.5772/intechopen.73123

Abstract

The prevalence of comorbid fibromyalgia syndrome in autoimmune rheumatic diseases is clinically significantly higher than is fibromyalgia syndrome in the general population. By increasing pain sensitivity and fatigue, it disproportionately inflates subjective signs and symptoms, thereby obfuscating composite indices used to measure biological disease activity, the degree of disability, and the quality of life. By modifying primary disease phenotype, it also interferes with diagnostic precision. This review documents its effects on rheumatoid arthritis, the spondyloarthropathies, and systemic lupus erythematosus; and offers a general remedial strategy.

Keywords: fibromyalgia, disease activity, diagnosis, outcomes

1. Introduction

Subjective symptoms such as patient global assessment of health (PtGA), fatigue, tenderness of joints at palpation (TJC), and even patient report of functional ability encountered in the evaluation of rheumatic diseases are very important not only because they reflect the individual patient's impression of disease activity and degree of disability, but also because patients place great faith in them [1]. Patients' estimation of pain, fatigue, and distress, which drive those subjective measures, is multidimensional, due to both biological disease activity as well as factors unrelated to disease-specific biological inflammation. Some of these factors include mechanical damage from comorbid osteoarthritis or disease-specific joint destruction and neuropathy from other disease, psychosocial factors, and even idiopathic poor sleep disorder. All of these factors can result in disproportionately higher subjective symptoms [2–4].

Composite indices such as the disease activity score (DAS) models are widely used to determine disease activity in clinical trials and everyday practice. Unfortunately, they may be misleading when used to evaluate apparent inflammatory activity in patients with comorbid chronic pain syndromes often coupled with psychological distress, which are synonymous with fibromyalgia syndrome (FMS). Comorbid FMS is associated with relative overestimation of subjective symptoms, which then inappropriately inflate the DAS models.

Fibromyalgia syndrome is comorbid in all rheumatic disease with prevalence as high as 25% in rheumatoid arthritis (RA), and 30% in systemic lupus erythematosus (SLE) and the spondyloarthropathies (SpA) [5–8]. The focus of this review will be on RA, SpA, and SLE.

1.1. Rheumatoid arthritis

In the past, when I spoke to rheumatologists about FMS, they often responded, "Why should I see patients with fibro? So many symptoms. And these patients with their personality disorders on top of anxiety and depression just wear me down. They're the worst."

The easy moral response might be, "Because these patients come to you for care, and you took an oath."

"I know, but why me?"

There are at least two other responses, both persuasive. The first appeals to the intellect. Fibromyalgia syndrome is a symptom complex at the severe end of a pain-distress spectrum [4, 9, 10]

It is a fascinating illness: a primary response to distress with demonstrated secondary process factors and dysfunction related to the endocrine [11] autonomic system[12], central nervous system [13], sleep quality [14], and arguably, even the immune system [15].

These process factors give rise to a plethora of symptoms including diffuse pain, fatigue, cognitive dysfunction, sleep disturbances, more severe morning stiffness, irritable bowel syndrome (IBS), headaches, Raynaud-like phenomenon, sicca symptoms, paresthesias, auditory dysfunction, bladder dysfunction, and among others [16–18].

The second is a practical response. The prevalence of FMS in the general population ranges from 2 to 8% [19–22]. As previously noted, the prevalence in rheumatic diseases is much higher. With practice, the clinician will become familiar with the FMS phenotype and be able to recognize it as a comorbidity in autoimmune rheumatic diseases. The reason that recognition is so important is, as we will see, that comorbid FMS, is often associated with psychological difficulties, that in concert with FMS can modify both the apparent phenotypic presentation and severity of clinical disease by inflating subjective symptoms.

For years, working at the Cleveland Clinic Foundation, a tertiary care practice, I evaluated RA patients who were referred because they were refractory to treatment, so-called "resistant arthritis" [23]. At final diagnosis, I could usually classify these patients into three categories:

http://dx.doi.org/10.5772/intechopen.73123

The majority either had only FMS, or did have RA, but the resistant symptoms were unrelated to RA and consistent with bursitis, tendinitis, OA, and especially FMS. In the third category, a very few had truly resistant RA disease activity.

At first blush, we might ask, "How is this possible?" When we learn that most rheumatologists no longer perform joint counts at office evaluation, we might better understand [24]. By failing to perform joint counts, they rely heavily on subjective symptoms such as the patient global assessment (PtGA) and patient evaluation of joint pain. Even when joint counts are included in the evaluation, mistakes can be made. Diffuse pain is by definition nonarticular, but can also include the joints [25–27], manifesting as a higher TJC. Comorbid FMS is also associated with increased duration and severity of morning stiffness, lower values for function measured as the Health Assessment Questionnaire-Disability Index (HAQ-DI), and the physical components of the SF-36 as well as diminished quality of life measured by the mental components of the same instrument [28, 29]. It is important to note a key diagnostic finding; in these reports, comorbid FMS did not usually associate with or obfuscate the swollen joint count (SJC) or acute phase reactants such as erythrocyte sedimentation rate (ESR), or c-reactive protein (CRP).

Comorbid FMS gives rise to enhanced pain sensitivity. The mechanism responsible for enhanced pain sensitivity is mediated in the central nervous system, facilitated by depression/anxiety [30–33]. In a cross-sectional analysis of a cohort of 305 FMS patients, depression showed the highest association with core FMS signs and symptoms [34]. The degree of depression showed a dose relationship with life-long numbers of TPs [35] and was responsible for the process of comorbid FMS in RA [36]. In a unique analysis using advanced Bayesian filtering of 247 diseases among 117,392 participants, depression was shown to be a primary comorbidity associated with FMS [37].

In summary, the effects of comorbid FMS on RA disease activity measures are many. It is associated with disproportionate elevation of PtGA and TJC [26, 28, 29, 38, 39]. The elevation of the subjective components of the DAS model indices inflates the total score. It is not surprising that in a recent analysis of change in disease status in patients with multiple comorbidities, PtGA best correlated with the other subjective variables, pain, and fatigue, which are also disproportionately elevated by comorbid FMS [40].

1.2. The spondyloarthropathies (SpA)

Diagnostic confusion is a larger problem in patients with SpA. An editorial reviewed the similarities between SpA and FMS, which included overlap of disease activity measures, found in patients with presumed enthesitis [41]. They asserted that FMS tender points (TPs) were anatomically located near or at enthesitis sites, which was confirmed in a separate study [8].

Because, as will be described, comorbid FMS disproportionately increases the Bath Ankylosing Spondylitis Disease Activity Index (BASDAI), Ankylosing Spondylitis Disease Activity Score (ASDAS), Bath Ankylosing Spondylitis Functional Index (BASFI), and Ankylosing Spondylitis

Quality of Life (ASQoL), it not only increases diagnostic confusion, but also interferes with accurate assessment of disease activity, disability, and quality of life. A strong case can be made for including FMS in the differential diagnosis of SpA.

Similarity between the two conditions was confirmed by Ablin and colleagues who approached the problem from the other perspective [42]. They carefully evaluated 99 patients who met 1990 ACR criteria for FMS, to determine whether some might also be classified as SpA. Ten patients fulfilled ASAS criteria for the diagnosis of axial SpA: eight of whom fulfilled the criteria based on MRI findings diagnostic of sacroiliitis, while two patients with negative MRI results fulfilled ASDAS criteria based on a positive HLA–B27 and the presence of SpA features.

One of the first studies to analyze phenotypic modification of ankylosing spondylitis by comorbid FMS was a cross-sectional study of 36 patients, 18 of each gender [43]. About 50% of women satisfied the criteria for comorbid FMS, whereas no males did. In this study, FMS correlated with the mean number of enthesitis sites. Higher BASDAI in women showed strong association with both the FMS incidence and a higher number of tender points. The perceived disability measured by BASFI was also significantly increased in patients with comorbid FMS. No association was found for the presence of FMS and the severity of physical findings or the ESR.

Interference with outcome measures was probably best demonstrated in an earlier study by Heikkila and colleagues [44]. They administered the BASDAI and BASFI, among other composite measures, to 24 women with SpA and 70 patients with FMS. The BASFI function demonstrated greater disability in the FMS group compared to SpA women.

If one is to rely on any one test in SpA with comorbid FMS, the ASDAS has been shown to be less obfuscated by comorbid FMS [45, 46]. These relationships to disease activity measures and a prevalence of FMS as high as 30% were largely confirmed by other studies [47–49]

The relatively high prevalence of FMS is not surprising, given the high prevalence of psychiatric problems in the SpA's estimated to be 40–50% [50]. When present, they similarly obfuscate measures of severity [50, 51]. "Patients with high risk for depression and anxiety had higher scores in BASDAI, BASFI, ASDAS-CRP, and also poorer scores for the pain visual analog scale (PVAS) and ankylosing spondylitis quality of life score" [51].

In summary, comorbid FMS complicates both diagnosis and estimation of disease activity in SpA. It follows that treatment decisions may also be obfuscated when FMS falsely inflates the BASDAI, PtGA, and BASFI [47]. This may lead to more frequent but inappropriate use of biologic agents, as it did in RA [52].

1.3. SLE

As discussed in the introduction, the prevalence of FMS in SLE has been reported to be at least as high as in RA ranging from five to 65% with a mean of ~30% [31, 53–65]. The core symptoms of FMS, diffuse pain, fatigue (low energy), cognitive difficulties, sleep disturbance, and depression will, of course, always be encountered in FMS comorbid disease.

Fatigue is present in at least 80% of patients with FMS. In a cross-sectional analysis of 100 SLE patients, fatigue correlated best with the presence of FMS, followed by depression and elevated PtGA [63]. In a very careful prospective blisibimod trial in SLE, improvement of fatigue was not clinically significant and correlated weakly only with SLE disease activity [66]. They hypothesized that, "...fatigue in SLE is multifactorial, with the 'non- SLE' component (including depression and fibromyalgia) less amenable to change during the trial."

Depression is a common comorbidity in unselected SLE cohorts ranging from 17 to 71% [31, 67]. The high prevalence of depression in SLE may help to explain the high prevalence of FMS. In a cohort study of 84 SLE patients, comorbid FMS was associated with anxiety and depression [60]. In a larger cohort of 276 SLE patients, the strongest association with both FMS and SLE/FM-like manifestations was a self-reported history of anxiety or affective disorder [65].

Quality of life (QoL) is closely associated with anxiety and depression in SLE [67]. In a study specifically designed to analyze health-related quality of life (HRQOL) in 138 SLE patients, all disease-specific HRQOL domains were significantly inversely correlated with disease activity, damage, depression, and the presence of FMS [59]. Comorbid FMS and depression was also shown to diminish QoL in two additional large SLE cohorts [68, 69].

Most analyses of health status in SLE have demonstrated that comorbid FMS is associated with increased disability [57, 60, 61, 65]. In a particularly important analysis, the number of tender points correlated with increasing disability demonstrating a dose effect [62].

Just as in RA and SpA, comorbid FMS modifies SLE disease activity measures. Sometimes, older papers are the best. In a study, published in 1994, the authors reported and analyzed differences in a cross-sectional analysis of 102 SLE patients [61]. "Twenty-two SLE patients (22%) met the American College of Rheumatology criteria for FMS, and another 24 (23%) had clinical FMS but did not meet the classification criteria," SLE patients with FMS and probable FMS (6–10 TPs) presented significantly higher Systemic Lupus Activity Measure (SLAM) scores. When the SLAM was modified by removing all subjective symptoms, neither category scored higher than SLE without FMS. This was also true for laboratory tests. Finally, patients who met criteria for FMS were much more likely to be unable to perform daily activities. By modifying components of disease severity composite indices, this early paper prefigured recent work in RA that employed the objective M-DAS or subjective DAS28-P [70, 71].

In the same year, Morand and colleagues reported the same phenomena in 87 SLE patients, 22, with FMS [57]. Manifestations of biological SLE disease activity, measured by the severity of specific organ system involvement, showed no difference between groups. The Systemic Lupus Activity Measurement scores were not significantly different. However, frequency of glucocorticoid use, antibodies to double-stranded DNA, the presence of at least four ACR criteria for SLE, and physician's global assessment (PhGA) were higher in the patients without FMS indicating more severe objective, biological disease in this subset. This analysis suggested that comorbid FMS in SLE can inappropriately increase the SLAM score.

Other indices appear to be relatively unaffected. In a cross-sectional analysis of 119 SLE patients, patients with FMS showed no effect on Systemic Lupus Erythematosus Activity

Index (SLEDAI) or Damage index, but did show poorer scores in all eight domains of the Short Form-36 [58]. The SLEDAI SLE disease activity score was also not influenced by FMS in another cohort of 100 SLE patients [63]. In another analysis of a much larger population of 458 SLE patients, comorbid FMS did not affect the 16-item SLE Symptom Scale [72]. These authors did not evaluate other composite indices.

Comorbid FMS signs and symptoms may also complicate the diagnostic process. For instance, when 149 presumed SLE patients with up to 5 years of disease duration were rigorously analyzed, 22 (14.3%) had only FMS with positive antinuclear antibodies (ANA) [73]. Depression, anxiety, fatigue, and sleep disturbance were the prominent symptoms in this group. Symptoms that indicated SLE included swollen joints, skin lesions, alopecia, renal disease, and serositis [72, 73].

The anti-nuclear antibody (ANA) test can be very confusing from the perspective of diagnosis. The high sensitivity of most and relatively low specificity of some ANA tests is problematic. Nonspecific (+) ANA in any titer can be found in roughly 30% of the general population, more likely in women and individuals 65 years and older [74–77]. Even titers as high as 1:320 are likely to be false positive in some settings, such as hospitalized patients [77]. The ANA is positive in low titer in at least 38% of individuals with FMS alone [78]. Furthermore, FMS patients with positive ANA tests are no more likely to have symptoms of autoimmune rheumatic disease than ANA-negative patients [53, 79], nor are they likely to later develop symptoms of an autoimmune disease in the future [80].

In summary, comorbid FMS inappropriately inflates some measures of SLE biological disease and, when patient with FMS have positive ANA testing, can interfere with diagnostic precision.

1.3.1. Parsing comorbid FMS: the RA models

Comorbid FMS in other diseases is not necessarily occult. It can be discovered both by clinical maneuvers and the use of validated questionnaires.

A very important study provided a basis for these maneuvers. The DAS28 was administered to 62 patients with RA and 26 patients with FMS alone [81]. Both groups had total scores consistent with moderate RA disease activity. But the component values were very different; the RA patients scored uniformly high for all components while the FMS cohort scored very high for the subjective TJC and PtGA and low on the objective SJC and ESR.

One clinical maneuver, which can be applied in RA, makes use of that observation; comorbid FMS disproportionally raises the TJC relative to the SJC. Comorbid FMS is likely to be present if the numerical difference is ≥7 when the SJC is subtracted from the TJC (39 Pollard). Alternatively, ratios of the TJC compared to the SJC may be used [30, 82]. In the third of these studies, depression, and by inference, pain, was shown to be a mediator of higher tender-to-swollen joint ratios [30].

To summarize, these last few studies have demonstrated that when the TJC is disproportionally higher than the SJC in RA: (1) comorbid pain amplification/FMS is a likely comorbidity, (2) biological RA disease activity, measured as the SJC and CRP/ESR, may be lower than

http://dx.doi.org/10.5772/intechopen.73123

indicated by the DAS28 composite score, and (3) joint count discordance should initiate a search for depression or other comorbidities that contribute to pain.

Two other RA studies created clinical maneuvers by modification of the DAS-model indices. In the first, the models were changed by removing the TJC and PTGA and adding the PhGA [70]. This "objective" DAS, termed the M-DAS, correlated better than the original DAS model with longitudinal magnetic resonance imaging (MRI) and radiographic outcome, providing better construct validity.

An alternative modification, DAS28-P, was created to reflect the proportion of the DAS28 derived from the PtGA and TJC [71]. This "subjective" index model correlated with higher articular and nonarticular pain pressure thresholds, fatigue, poorer mental health, and most importantly, the presence of FMS.

Another instrument that has been specifically designed to recognize FMS alone or as a comorbid condition is the Polysymptomatic Distress Score (PSD) [83]. This instrument incorporates questions about pain and core symptoms of FMS, and has been demonstrated to measure comorbid FMS prevalence and severity in RA [84].

In summary, both comorbid FMS and depression disproportionately inflate symptoms of pain and fatigue which, in turn, amplify PtGA and other subjective patient-report-only indices. These disproportionately higher subjective components then raise the total score of the composite index, falsely indicating higher biological disease. Biological disease activity is not worsened by comorbid FMS; it is only the measures, the ratings, that are obfuscated by FMS.

1.3.2. Remedies

One appropriate approach to the comorbid FMS problem in all of these diseases might be to construct two separate indices: one comprised of symptoms that arise from patient perceptions of pain, distress, and fatigue (PtGA, TJC, number of enthesitis sites, disability) and the other measures of objective inflammatory burden (acute phase reactants, SJC) and target organ damage. If these two separate indices are discordant, those symptoms and signs of FMS or autoimmune biological disease activity are treated separately and differently. Treatments for FMS and psychological disorders versus biological disease activity are distinctly different. This strategy should limit potential inappropriate over-treatment of the primary disease and provide better control of pain, distress, and fatigue, factors that are not necessarily intrinsically related to biological disease activity.

Acknowledgements

None. I am the sole author

Ethical approval and patient

Neither Individual patients nor their medical records were involved in this literature review.

Funding

This work was not funded.

Disclosure statement

I currently work as an independent medical biotechnical consultant, and in the past, have consulted for Crescendo Bioscience. and Pfizer.

Contributorship

I am the sole author and 100% contributor.

Data sharing statement

None

Author details

William S. Wilke

Address all correspondence to: wswilkemd@gmail.com

Rheumatology Department, Cleveland Clinic Orthopedic and Rheumatology Institute, Cleveland, Ohio, USA

References

[1] Carr A, Hewlett S, Hughes R, Mitchell H, Ryan S, Carr M, et al. Rheumatology outcomes: The patient's perspective. Journal of Rheumatology. 2003;**30**:880-883

[2] Lee YC, Bingham CO, Edwards RR, et al. Pain sensitization is associated with disease activity in rheumatoid arthritis patients: A cross-sectional study. Arthritis Care Research (Hobogen). Dec 2017;**69**(12):1871-1877. DOI: 10.1002/acr.23266. [Epub ahead of print]

[3] Matcham F, Ali S, Irving K, et al. Are depression and anxiety associated with disease activity in rheumatoid arthritis? A prospective study. BMC Musculoskeletal Disorders. 2016;**17**(155). The authors analyzed the effects of depression and anxiety

on the DAS28 in 56 RA patients followed prospectively for 1 year. "After adjusting for age, gender, disease duration and baseline tender joint count and patient global assessment respectively, higher levels of depression and anxiety at baseline were associated with increased tender joint count and patient global assessment scores at 1-year follow-up."

[4] Wolfe F. The relation between tender points and fibromyalgia symptom variables: Evidence that fibromyalgia is not a discrete disorder. Annals of the Rheumatic Disorders. 1997;**56**:268-271

[5] Atzeni F, Cazzola M, Benucci M, et al. Chronic widespread pain in the spectrum of rheumatological diseases. Best Practice Research and Clinic Rheumatology. 2011;**25**:165-171. FMS (1990 ACR) is often associated with other diseases that act as confounding and aggravating factors, including primary Sjögren's syndrome (pSS), systemic lupus erythematosus (SLE) and rheumatoid arthritis (RA). It has been reported to coexist in 25% of patients with RA, 30% of patients with SLE and 50% of patients with pSS. It is associated with diminished QoL

[6] Haliloglu S, Carlioglu A, Akdeiz D, et al. Fibromyalgia in patients with other rheumatic diseases: Prevalence and relationship with disease activity. Rheumatology Introduction. 2014;**34**:1275-1280. The prevalence of FMS in patients with rheumatologic diseases was found to be 6.6% for RA, 13.4% for SLE, 12.6% for AS, 10.1% for OA, 5.7% for BD, 7.1% for FMF, 12% for SS, 25% for vasculitis, 1.4% for gout, and 6.9% for PMR. Increased pain, physical limitations, and fatigue may be interpreted as increased activity of these diseases, and a common treatment option is the prescription of higher doses of biologic agents or corticosteroids

[7] El-Rabbat SM, Mahmoud NK, Gheita TA. Clinical significance of fibromyalgia syndrome in different rheumatic diseases: Relation to disease activity and quality of life. Reumatology Clinical. April 11, 2017. Pii: S1699-258X(17)30048-7. Doi: 10.1016/j.reuma.2017.02.008. [Epub ahead of print]. 160 patients (50 RA, 50 SLE, 30 SSc and 30 BD) and matched corresponding healthy controls were included. Disease activity was assessed using disease activity score in 28 joints (DAS28) for RA, SLE Disease Activity index (SLEDAI), modified Rodnan skin score for SSc and BD Current Activity Form (BDCAF). The QoL was also recorded. In the RA, SLE, SSc and BD patients, FMS was found in 14, 18, 6.67 and 3.33% respectively compared to 2.1, 3, 3.3 and 0% in their corresponding controls. In RA DAS was significantly higher and Quol lower. In SLE the SSscale of the PSD correlated with the SLEDAI

[8] Roussou E, Ciurtin C. Clinical overlap between fibromyalgia tender points and enthesitis sites in patients with spondyloarthritis who present with inflammatory back pain. Clinical and Experimenal Rheumatology. 2012;**30**(Suppl 74):24-30

[9] Croft P, Rigby AS, Boswell R, et al. The prevalence of chronic widespread pain in the general population. Journal of Rheumatology. 1993;**20**:710-713

[10] Wessely S, Nimnuan C, Sharpe M. Functional somatic syndromes: One or many? Lancet. 1999;**354**:936-939

[11] Tak LM, Cleare AJ, Ormel J, et al. Meta-analysis and meta-regression of hypothalamic–pituitary–adrenal axis activity in functional somatic disorders. Biological Psychology. May 2011;**87**(2):183-194

[12] Martinez-Martinez LA, Mora T, Vargas A, et al. Sympathetic nervous system dysfunction in fibromyalgia, chronic fatigue syndrome, irritable bowel syndrome, and interstitial cystitis. A review of case–control studies. Journal of Clinical Rheumatology. 2014;**20**:146-150

[13] Kim H, Kim J, Loggia ML, et al. Fibromyalgia is characterized by altered frontal and cerebellar structural covariance brain networks. Neurolimage: Clinical. 2015;**7**:667-677

[14] Choy E. The role of sleep in pain and fibromyalgia. Nat Rev Rheumatol. Advance online publication Sep 2015;**11**(9):513-520. DOI: 10.1038/nrrhuem.2015.56

[15] Uceyler N, Hauser W, Sommer C. Systematic review with meta-analysis: Cytokines in fibromyalgia syndrome. BMC Musculoskeletal Disorders. 2011;**12**:245 (15 of 15)

[16] Bradley LA, Alarcon GS. Miscellaneous rheumatic diseases. In: Kopman WJ, Moreland LW, editors. Arthritis and Allied Conditions. 15th ed. Philadelphia: Lipincott Williams & Wilkins; 2005. pp. 1869-1910

[17] Wolfe F, Ross K, Anderson J, Russell IJ, Hebert L. The prevalence and characteristics of fibromyalgia in the general population. Arthritis and Rheumatism. 1995;**38**(1):19-28

[18] Clauw DJ. Fibromyalgia: Update on mechanisms and management. Journal of Clinical Rheumatology. 2007;**13**:102-109

[19] Wolfe F, Smythe HA, Yunus MB, et al. The American College of rheumatology 1990 criteria for the classification of fibromyalgia. Report of the Multicenter Criteria Committee. Arthritis and Rheumatism. 1990;**33**:160-172

[20] McBeth J, Jones K. Epidemiology of chronic musculoskeletal pain. Best Practice and Research: Clinical Rheumatology. 2007;**21**(3):403-425

[21] Vincent A, Lahr BD, Wolfe F, et al. Prevalence of fibromyalgia: A population-based study in Olmsted County, Minnesota, utilizing the Rochester Epidemiology Project. Arthritis Care Research (Hoboken). 2013;**65**(5):786-792

[22] Phillips K, Clauw DJ. Central pain mechanisms in the rheumatic diseases: Future directions. Arthritis and Rheumatism. 2013;**65**(2):291-302

[23] Wilke WS, Duna GF. When resistant RA calls for aggressive intervention. Journal of Musculoskeletal Medicine. 1994;**11**:33-37

[24] Pincus T, Segurado OG. Most visits of most patients with rheumatoid arthritis to most rheumatologists do not include a formal quantitative joint count. Annals of the Rheumatic Diseases. 2006;**65**:820-822

[25] Leeb BF, Haindl PM, Maktari A, et al. Disease activity score-28 values differ considerably depending on patient's pain perception and sex. Journal of Rheumatology. 2007;**34**:2382-2387

[26] Pollard LC, Ibrahim F, Choy EH, Scott DL. Pain thresholds in rheumatoid arthritis: The effects of tender point counts and disease duration. Journal of Rheumatology. 2012;**39**(1):28-31

[27] Urrows S, Affleck G, Tennen H, Higgins P. Unique clinical and psychological correlates of fibromyalgia tender points and joint tenderness in rheumatoid arthritis. Arthritis and Rheumatism. 1994 October;**37**(10):1513-1520

[28] Wolfe F. Pain extent and diagnosis: Development and validation of the regional pain scale in 12,799 patients with rheumatic disease. Journal of Rheumatology. 2003;**30**:369-378

[29] Coury F, Rossat A, Tebib A, et al. Rheumatoid arthritis and fibromyalgia: A frequent unrelated association complicating disease management. Rheumatology. 2009;**36**:58-62

[30] Schweinhardt P, Kalk N, Wartolowska KK, et al. Investigation into the neural correlates of emotional augmentation of chronic pain. Neuroimage. 2008;**40**:759-766. This publication also provides insight into a potential mechanism, namely that the central nervous system mediates a higher tender-to swollen joint count phenomenon The relationships of a dichotomized Beck Depression Index (BDI) either low or high, to standard joint pressure evoked tenderness and functional magnetic resonance imaging were analyzed in 20 RA patients. The authors demonstrated that BDI categories, higher tender-to-swollen joint counts and activity in pain processing regions of the brain all correlated. C-reactive protein was not correlate with these three measures. This study identified depression, and by inference, pain as a mediator of higher tender-to-swollen joint ratios

[31] Wolfe F, Michaud K, Li T, Katz RS. Chronic conditions and health problems in rheumatic diseases: Comparisons with rheumatoid arthritis, noninflammatory rheumatic disorders, systemic lupus erythematosus, and fibromyalgia. Journal of Rheumatology. 2010;**37**:305-315

[32] Fifield J, Tennen H, Reisine S, McQuillan J. Depression and the long-term risk of pain, fatigue, and disability in patients with rheumatoid arthritis. Arthritis and Rheumatism. 1998;**41**:1851-1857

[33] Schieir O, Thombs BD, Hudson M, et al. Symptoms of depression predict the trajectory of pain among patients with early inflammatory arthritis: A path analysis approach to assessing change. Journal of Rheumatology. 2009;**36**:231-239

[34] Gota CE, Kaouk S, Wilke WS. The impact of depressive and bipolar symptoms on socioeconomic status, core symptoms, function and severity of fibromyalgia. International Journal of Rheumatology. Mar 2017;**20**(3):326-339. DOI: 10.1111/1756-185X.12603. [Epub ahead of print]

[35] Brown D, Mulvey M, Cordingly L, et al. The relationship between psychological distress and multiple tender points across the adult lifespan. Archives of Gerontology and Geriatrics. 2016;**63**:102-107

[36] Kapoor SR, Hider SL, Brownfield A, et al. Fibromyalgia in patients with rheumatoid arthritis: Driven by depression or joint damage? Clinical and Experimental Rheumatology. 2011;**29**(Suppl. 69):S88-S91

[37] Marx P, Antal P, Bolgar B, et al. Comorbidities in the diseasome are more apparent than real: What Bayesian filtering reveals about the comorbidities of depression. PLoS Computational Biology. 2017;**13**(6) e1005487

[38] Ton E, Bakker MF, Verstappen SM, et al. Look beyond the disease activity score of 28 joints (DAS28): Tender points influence the DAS28 in patients with rheumatoid arthritis. Journal of Rheumatology. January 2012;**39**(1):22-27. The authors conducted a cross-sectional analysis of 200 consecutive RA patients with active disease. In 15% of patients, the tender point count (TPC) was ≥11, in 12% 6-10, in 30% 1-5, and in 43% zero. The TPC was positively associated with the DAS, TJC and PtGAThe authors conducted a cross-sectional analysis of 200 consecutive RA patients with active disease. In 15% of patients, the tender point count (TPC) was ≥11, in 12% 6-10, in 30% 1-5, and in 43% zero. The TPC was positively associated with the DAS, TJC and PtGA

[39] Pollard LC, Kingsley GS, Chow EH, Scott DL. Fibromyalgic rheumatoid arthritis and disease assessment. Rheumatology. 2010;**49**:924-928. The authors analyzed 205 RA patients in two cross-sectional cohorts. Thirty (14.6%) patients met 1990 American College of Rheumatology (ACR) Criteria for FMS. Patients who met the criterion TJC minus the SJC ≥ 7 identified as ACR FMS with sensitivity of ~76% and specificity of ~89%. Both criteria identified patients with greater pain, fatigue, HAQ disability, PtGA and DAS28 compared to patients without FMS. The SJC and ESR were not different between cohorts

[40] Radner H, Yoshida K, Tedeschi S, et al. Different rating of global rheumatoid arthritis disease activity in rheumatoid arthritis patients with multiple morbidities. Arthritis Rheumatology. 2007;**69**:720-727

[41] Wendling D, Prati C. Spondyloarthritis and fibromyalgia: Interfering association or differential diagnosis. Clinical Rheumatology. 2016;**35**:2141-2143

[42] Ablin JN, Eshed I, Berman M, et al. Prevalence of axial spondyloarthritis among patients with fibromyalgia: A magnetic resonance imaging study with application of the assessment of spondyloArthritis international society classification criteria. Arthritis Care Research. 2017;**69**:724-729

[43] Aloush V, Ablin JN, Reitblat T, Caspi D, Elkayam O. Fibromyalgia in women with ankylosing spondylitis. Rheumatology International. 2007;**27**:865-868

[44] Heikkila S, Ronni S, Kautiainen HJ, Kauppi M. Functional impairment in spondyloarthropathy and fibromyalgia. Journal of Rheumatology. 2002;**29**:1415-1419

[45] Wach J, Letroublon M-C, Coury F, Tebib JG. Fibromyalgia in spondiloarthritis: Effect on disease in clinical practice. Journal of Rheumatology. 2016;**43**:2056-2063

[46] Salaffi F, De Angelis R, Carotti M, Gutierrez M, Sarzi-Puttini P, Atzeni F. Fibromyalgia in patients with axial spondyloarthritis: Epidemiological profile and effect on measures of disease activity. Rheumatology International. 2014;**34**:1103-1110

[47] Bello N, Etcheto A, Beal C, et al. Evaluation of the impact of fibromyalgia in disease activity and treatment effect in spondyloarthritis. Arthritis Research and Therapy. 2016;**18**:42. DOI: 10.1186/s13075-016-0943-z

[48] Azevedo VF, Paiva Edos S, Felippe LR, Moreira RA. Occurrence of fibromyalgia in patients with ankylosing spondylitis. Revista Brasileira Reumatologia. 2010;**50**:646-650

[49] Almodóvar R, Carmona L, Zarco P, Collantes E, González C, Mulero J, et al. Fibromyalgia in patients with ankylosing spondylitis: Prevalence and utility of the measures of activity, function and radiological damage. Clinical and Experimental Rheumatology. 2010;**28**(Suppl 63):S33-S39

[50] Durmus D, Sarisoy G, Alaya G, et al. Psychiatric symptoms in ankylosing spondylitis: Their relationship with disease activity, functional capacity, pain and fatigue. Comprehensive Psychiatry. 2015;**62**:170-177

[51] Kilic G, Kilic E, Ozgocmen S. Relationship between psychiatric status, self-reported outcome measures, and clinical parameters in axial Spondyloarthritis. Medicine. 2014;**93**(29):e337

[52] Lage-Hansen PR, Chrysidis S, Lage-Hansen M, Hougaard A, Ejstrup L, Amris K. Concomitant fibromyalgia in rheumatoid arthritis is associated with the more frequent use of biological therapy: A cross-sectional study. Scandinavian Journal of Rheumatology. 2015;**16**:1-4

[53] Zonana-Nacach A, Alarcon GS, Reveille JD, et al. Clinical features of ANA-positive and vANA-negative fibromyalgia patients. Journal of Clinical Rheumatology. 1998;**4**:52-56

[54] Handa R, Aggarwal P, Wali JP, Wig N, Dwivedi SN. Fibromyalgia in Indian patients with SLE. Lupus. 1998;**7**:475-478

[55] Valencia-Flores M, Cardiel MH, Santiago V, et al. Prevalence and factors associated with fibromyalgia in Mexican patients with systemic lupus erythematosus. Lupus. 2004;**13**:4-10

[56] Neumann L, Buskila D. Epidemiology of fibromyalgia. Current Pain and Headache Reports. 2003;**7**:362-368. A review. Chronic widespread pain, the cardinal symptom of FMS, is common in the general population, with comparable prevalence rates of 7.3-12.9% across different countries

[57] Morand EF, Miller MH, Whittingham S, Littlejohn GO. Fibromyalgia syndrome and disease activity in systemic lupus erythematosus. Lupus. 1994;**3**:187, 191. "We conclude that FS is prevalent in individuals with SLE and does not affect disease expression but may interfere with the rating of disease activity (SLAM)"

[58] Gladman DD, Urowitz MB, Gough J. MacKinnon: Fibromyalgia is a major contributor to quality of life in lupus. Journal of Rheumatology. 1997;**24**:2145-2148. Analyzed 119 SLE patients. FMS prevalence 21%. No effect on SLEDAI or Damage index, but was highly correlated with all 8 domains of the SF-36

[59] Etchegaray-Moralis I, Mendez-Martinez S, Jimenez-Hernandez C, et al. Factors associated with health-related quality of life in Mexican Lupus patients using the LupusQol. Plos One. 2017 January 23;**12**(1):e0170209). DOI: 10.1371/journal.pone.0170209. eCollection 2017 A cross-sectional study was conducted in 138 women fulfilling the 1997 ACR

classification criteria for SLE. Associations:19.6% with FMS with SLE disease activity, damage, fibromyalgia and depression and with poor HRQOL in this sample of Mexican SLE patients

[60] Torrente-Segarra V, Carbonell Abello J, Castro Oreiro S, Manresa Domnguez JM. Association between fibromyalgia and psychiatric disorders in systemic lupus erythematosus. Clinical Experimental and Rheumatology. 2010;**28**(Suppl. 63):S22-S26. Thirty patients were diagnosed with FMS (35.7%), 16 (19%) had clinical signs of depressive symptoms (DS) and 30 (35.7%) had clinical signs of anxiety symptoms (AS). They found a statistically significant association between FMS and AS ($p < 0.001$), and between FM and DS ($p < 0.001$) Higher SF-12 physical component and mental component scores were observed in FMS group compared to non-FMS group ($p < 0.001$)

[61] Middleton GD, JE MF, Lipsky PE. The prevalence and clinical impact of fibromyalgia in systemic lupus erythematosus. Arthritis and Rheumatism. 1994;**37**:1181-1188. The paper reported a cross-sectional analysis of 102 patients from a public hospital SLE clinic. Information was obtained on symptoms of FMS, disability, tender points, pain thresholds, and SLE disease activity. Twenty-two SLE patients (22%) met the American College of Rheumatology criteria for FMS, and another 24 (23%) had clinical FMS but did not meet the classification criteria. This group was much more likely to be unable to perform daily activities but did not differ in measures of SLE activity General Health, Social Function, and overall Physical Component Functioning (CS) scores underscoring the need for effective treatments for FM in SLE. Atorvastatin did not have any apparent effect on HRQOL. SELENA-SLEDAI did not correlate with PCS

[62] Akkasilpa S, Goldman D, Magder LS, Petri M. Number of fibromyalgia tender points is associated with health status in patients with systemic lupus erythematosus. Journal of Rheumatology. 2005;**32**:48-50. In this SLE cohort 17.3% had at least 11tender points (TP). There were significant associations between TPs and HAQ. There was also a strong association between the number of TPs and health status. The number of TPs, and not just the presence/absence of FMS, iwas associated with diminished health status (HAQ-DI) in SLE

[63] Wang B, Gladman DD, Urowitz MB. Fatigue in lupus not correlated with disease activity. Journal of Rheumatology. 1998;**25**:892-895. Analyzed 100 SLE patients, 21% with FMS. Fatigue associated with FMS, depression and SF-20, but not SLEDAI

[64] Valencia-Flores M, Cardiel MH, Santiago V, Resendiz M, Castano VA, Negrete O, et al. Prevalence and factors associated with fibromyalgia in Mexican patients with systemic lupus erythematosus. Lupus. 2004;**13**(1):4-10

[65] Friedman AW, Tewi MB, Ahn C, et al. Systemic lupus erythematosus in three ethnic groups: XV. Prevalence and correlates of fibromyalgia. Lupus. 2003;**12**:274-279. Fibromyalgia syndrome was present in 14 patients (5%; 9/92 Caucasians (C), 4/109 African Americans (AA), 1/65 Hispanics (H)) and FM/FM-like manifestations in 35 (13%; 16 C, 9 AA, 10 H). By stepwise logistic regression analyses, the strongest association

with both FM and SLE/FM-like manifestations was a self-reported history of anxiety or affective disorder (P = 0.0237, OR = 4.6 and P = 0.0068, OR = 3.4, respectively). Poorer self-reported physical functioning was associated with the SLE/FM-like phenotype (P = 0.0443, OR = 0.96). Clinical measures of disease activity, disease damage, specific organ dysfunction, sociodemographic factors and serologic features were not correlated with FMS in this early SLE cohort

[66] Petri M, Martin RS, Scheinberg MA, et al. Assessments of fatigue and disease activity in patients with systemic lupus erythematosus enrolled in the phase 2 clinical trial with blisibimod. Lupus. 2017;**26**:2737. "In these analyses, patient-reported fatigue in SLE as quantified by the FACIT-Fatigue instrument was statistically significantly but weakly correlated with disease activity (range of observed Spearman coefficients –0.13 to –0.31 at Week 24)." However, the low correlation coefficients suggest that these relationships between FACIT Fatigue are not clinically significant. We hypothesize that fatigue in SLE is multifactorial, with the 'non-SLE' component (including depression and fibromyalgia) less amenable to change during the trial."

[67] Shen B, Feng G, Tang W, Huang X, Yan H, He Y, et al. The quality of life in Chinese patients with systemic lupus erythematosus is associated with disease activity and psychiatric disorders: A path analysis. Clinical Experimental and Rheumatology. 2014;**32**:101-107. Data were collected from 170 SLE patients and 210 healthy individuals. Depression, anxiety and disease activity contributed to HRQoL both directly and indirectly through other factors. Socioeconomic factors such as education, income/family and work status, however, did not contribute directly to HRQoL

[68] Abu-Shakra M, Mader R, Langevitz P, Friger M, Codish S, Neumann L, et al. Quality of life in systemic lupus erythematosus: A controlled study. Journal of Rheumatology. 1999;**26**:306-309

[69] Kiani AN, Strand V, Fang H, et al. Predictors of self-reported health-related quality of life in systemic lupus erythematosus. Rheumatology. 2013;**52**:1651-1657. This paper reported data from the longitudinal atorvastin study. Among 200 SLE patients FMS was independently associated with poorer HRQOL in most domains and was significantly associated with lower Physical Functioning, Role Physical and Bodily Pain

[70] Baker JF, Conaghan PG, Smolen JS, et al. Development and validation of modified disease activity scores in rheumatoid arthritis superior correlation with magnetic resonance imaging–detected synovitis and radiographic progression. Arthritis and Rheumatology. 2014;**66**(4):794-802. This is a land mark paper that demonstrated construct validity deficiencies of PtGA and TJC. In this 52-week prospective analysis of 186 patients who participated in the GO-BEFORE and GO-FORWARD clinical trials, the authors compared the correlation of a modified version of the disease activity score with 28 joints and c-reactive protein (M-DAS28-CRP) (TJC, PtGA removed and PhGA substituted), and the original DAS28-CRP with joint damage. This M-DAS28 correlated better with longitudinal magnetic resonance imaging (MRI) and radiographic outcome at 26 and 52 weeks. Similar modification of the Simplified Disease Activity Index and the Clinical

Disease Activity Index (CDAI) essentially replicated the M-DAS28 findings. The TJC and PtGA demonstrate poor construct validity, which diminished the validity of DAS28. According to the authors, "These findings speak to the subjectivity of the TJC28 and the patient global assessment, each of which can be high in subjects with relatively low levels of inflammation."

[71] Joharatnam N, McWilliams DF, Wilson D, et al. A cross sectional study of pain sensitivity, disease activity assessment, mental health and fibromyalgia status in rheumatoid arthritis. Arthritis Research. January 20, 2015;**17**:11. DOI: 10.1186/s13075-015-0525-5. This was an analysis of 50 participants with long-standing RA with DAS28 score > 3.1 (47). Fibromyalgia, defined by the Polysymptomatic Distress score was common at 48%. Patients with higher DAS28 and DAS-P (using only the TJC and PtGA) had higher sensitivity to pressure-induced pain and prevalence of FMS. The authors suggested that measures of mental health should be obtained in patients with high DAS28 scores. In a prior analysis by the same group, the DAS-P associated with current pain and predicted poorer prognosis

[72] Wolfe F, Petri M, Alarcon GS, et al. Fibromyalgia, Systemic Lupus Erythematosus (SLE), and Evaluation of SLE Activity. Journal of Rheumatology. 2009;**36**:82-88

[73] Calvo-Alen J, Bastian HM, Straaton KV, et al. Identification of patient subsets among those presumptively diagnosed with, referred, and/or followed up for systemic lupus erythematosus at a large tertiary care center. Arthritis Rheumatology. 1995;**38**:1475-1484. When the ACR criteria for SLE were used to determine eligibility for lupus studies, a group of patients with a previous diagnosis of SLE were classified into one of three categories: 1) SLE by the American College of Rheumatology (ACR; formerly, the American Rheumatism Association) criteria, 2) clinical SLE but not meeting 4 of the ACR criteria, or 3) fibromyalgia-like manifestations with antinuclear antibody (ANA) positivity. There were 90 patients in the first group (criteria), 22 in the second group (clinical), and 37 in the third group (fibromyalgia-like)

[74] De Vlam K, De Keyser F, Verbruggen G, et al. Detection and identification of antinuclear autoantibodies in the serum of normal blood donors. Clinical and Experimental Rheumatology. 1993;**11**:393-397

[75] Craig WY, Ledue TB, Johnson AM, Ritchie RF. The distribution of antinuclear antibody titers in "normal" children and adults. Journal of Rheumatology. 1999;**26**:914-919

[76] Tan EM, Feltkamp TEW, Smolen JS, et al. Range of antinuclear antibodies in "healthy" individuals. Arthritis and Rheumatism. 1997;**40**:1601-1611

[77] Slater CA, Davis RB, Shmerling RH. Antinuclear antibody testing. A study of clinical utility. Archives of Internal Medicine. 1996;**156**:1421-1425

[78] Suarez-Almazor ME, Gonzalez-Lopez L, Gamez-Nava JI, Belseck E, Kendall CJ, Davis P. Utilization and predictive value of laboratory tests in patients referred to rheumatologists by primary care physicians. Journal of Rheumatology. October 1998;**25**(10):1980-1985

[79] Vaile JH, Dyke L, Kherani R, Johnston C, Higgins T, Russell AS. Is high titer ANA specific for connective tissue disease? Clinical and Experimental Rheumatology. 2000;**18**:433-438

[80] Kötter I, Neuscheler D, Günaydin I, Wernet D, Rl K. Is there a predisposition for the development of autoimmune diseases in patients with fibromyalgia? Retrospective analysis with long term follow-up. Rheumatology International. 2007;**27**:1031-1039. The risk of CTD was not increased in FMS. The detection of ANA does not predict the development of CTD

[81] Leeb BF, Andel J, Sautner T, Nothnagl T, Rintelen B. The DAS28 in rheumatoid arthritis and fibromyalgia patients. Rheumatology. 2004;**43**(12):1504-1507

[82] Kristensen LE, Bliddal H, Christensen R, et al. Is swollen to tender joint count ratio a new and useful clinical marker for biologic drug response in rheumatoid arthritis? Results from a Swedish cohort. Arthritis Care Research. 2014;**66**:173-179. In this large study, 2507 RA patients individuals were assigned to three categories determined by the ratio of swollen-to-tender joints (STR): low (<0.5); moderate (0.5 ≤ STR ≥ 1.0); and high (>1.0) (39). The percentage of ACR 50 response to initial anti-tumor necrosis-alpha therapy was evaluated among the three categories. Patients with moderate and high STR experienced significantly higher absolute responses than low STR patients. One interpretation of these findings posited that RA patients with low STR (higher TJCs than SJCs) have milder objective biological RA disease activity, therefore less absolute numerical inflammation and so will appear to respond less well to "anti-inflammatory" treatment

[83] Wolfe F, Clauw DJ, FitzCharles MA, Goldenberg DL, Katz RS, Mease P, et al. The American College of Rheumatology preliminary diagnostic criteria for fibromyalgia and measurement of symptom severity. Arthritis Care Research (Hoboken). 2010;**62**:600-610

[84] Wolfe F, Michaud K, Busch RE, et al. Polysymptomatic distress in patients with rheumatoid arthritis: Understanding disproportionate response and its spectrum. Arthritis Care Research. 2014;**66**:1465-1471. In a very important paper, Wolfe and coworkers analyzed 300 RA patients prior to therapy using the PSD scale. Among those RA patients, 123 (41%) had widespread pain and 61 (20.3%) met 2010 Preliminary Criteria for FMS. As the PSD score increased, all variables; CDAI, and individual composite measures, as well as pain, Health Assessment Questionnaire-II (HAQ-II), and the Patient Activity Scale-II (PAS-II) also increased. This increase was most pronounced in the more "subjective" measures including pain, TJC, PtGA, HAQ-II and PAS-II. Even "objective" variables, including PhGA and the SJC were increased, but less dramatically. Alternatively, low PSD scores were associated with discordantly lower values. The authors concluded that, "These findings indicate that DAS model composite index disease activity measures have low precision." The authors further opined that, "These data suggest a certain futility in using a single composite measure to evaluate RA illness. Inflammation and joint damage are just that; they are not pain or suffering or tender joints